MORE PRAISE FOR

Home for Dinner

"There are magical opportunities for tenderness, courage, healing, laughter— and almost everything else it means to be human—when the people we love come together to eat the food we love. This remarkably wise, engaging, lovely book is an invaluable guide for all of us in creating this magic. Give yourself the pleasure of reading it and join The Family Dinner Project."
—Richard Weissbourd, Faculty Director of the Human Development and Psychology Program, Harvard Graduate School of Education

"Anne Fishel's warmth, wisdom, and humor are the ingredients that make this book such a delight to read. I recommend it to anyone who has the opportunity to eat with others—new couples, parents, and grandparents— because while it delights you, it will also convince you that we can and should eat well and do it together."
—Paula Rauch, MD, Director, Marjorie E. Korff PACT Program (Parenting At a Challenging Time); Program Director, Family Support and Outreach, Red Sox Foundation/ MGH Home Base Program; Associate Professor of Psychiatry, Harvard Medical School

"Anne Fishel's book *Home for Dinner* is simply delicious. It is filled with helpful suggestions about family dinners rich with fun and good food. The book is packed with recipes for food, conversation, and community building. Anyone can read it, enjoy the completely engaging style, and learn to reap the health, mental health, and family benefits of family dinners."
—John Sargent, MD, Professor of Psychiatry and Pediatrics, Tufts University School of Medicine

"Anne Fishel serves up a sumptuous banquet of compelling science, clinical wisdom, family psychology, delicious recipes, and a lively, personal style into a single book that will nourish families in mind, body, and spirit."
—Martha B. Straus, Ph.D., Professor of Clinical Psychology, Antioch University New England; author of *Adolescent Girls in Crisis: Intervention and Hope*

"*Home for Dinner* offers a feast of insights, hands-on advice, and mouthwatering recipes that will equip readers to turn the necessity of eating into an opportunity for growing family relationships, building children's intelligence and social skills, and nourishing healthy bodies and minds. Research-based, story-sprinkled, and supremely practical—an enlightening read."
—Abigail Carroll, author of *Three Squares: The Invention of the American Meal*

HOME

FOR

DINNER

Mixing Food, Fun, and Conversation
for a Happier Family
and Healthier Kids

Anne K. Fishel, Ph.D.

FOREWORD BY

Michael Thompson, Ph.D.

◢AMACOM

AMERICAN MANAGEMENT ASSOCIATION

New York • Atlanta • Brussels • Chicago • Mexico City • San Francisco
Shanghai • Tokyo • Toronto • Washington, D.C.

Bulk discounts available. For details visit:
www.amacombooks.org/go/specialsales
Or contact special sales:
Phone: 800-250-5308
Email: specialsls@amanet.org
View all the AMACOM titles at: www.amacombooks.org
American Management Association: www.amanet.org

This publication is designed to provide accurate and authoritative information in regard to the subject matter covered. It is sold with the understanding that the publisher is not engaged in rendering legal, accounting, or other professional service. If legal advice or other expert assistance is required, the services of a competent professional person should be sought.

Library of Congress Cataloging-in-Publication Data

Fishel, Anne K.
  Home for dinner : mixing food, fun, and conversation for a happier family and healthier kids / Anne K. Fishel, Ph.D. ; foreword by Michael Thompson, Ph.D.
     pages cm
  Includes bibliographical references and index.
  ISBN 978-0-8144-3370-6 (pbk.) — ISBN 0-8144-3370-7 (pbk.) — ISBN 978-0-8144-3371-3 (ebook)
  1. Families.   2. Dinners and dining—Social aspects.   3. Dinners and dining—Psychological aspects.   I. Title.
  HQ734.F448 2014
  306.85—dc23   2014036476

About AMA
American Management Association (www.amanet.org) is a world leader in talent development, advancing the skills of individuals to drive business success. Our mission is to support the goals of individuals and organizations through a complete range of products and services, including classroom and virtual seminars, webcasts, webinars, podcasts, conferences, corporate and government solutions, business books, and research. AMA's approach to improving performance combines experiential learning—learning through doing—with opportunities for ongoing professional growth at every step of one's career journey.

Printing number

10 9 8 7 6 5 4 3 2 1

To my sons, Gabe and Joe,
and
To my husband, Chris,
For all our dinners at home

Contents

Foreword by Michael Thompson, Ph.D.   ix

Acknowledgments   xiii

PART ONE   SETTING THE TABLE

1. Welcome to the Table   3

2. What's So Great About Family Dinners?   12

3. One Size Dinner Doesn't Fit All Ages   24

**PART TWO   THE MAIN COURSE: FOOD, FUN,
                AND CONVERSATION**

4. Tips for Healthy Eating   49

5. Play with Your Food   77

6. Table Talk That Goes Beyond "How Was Your Day?"   103

7. Telling Stories to Promote Empathy, Self-Esteem, Resilience, and Enjoyment   119

PART THREE   SERVING IT FORWARD: USING DINNER TO MAKE CHANGE IN YOUR FAMILY AND BEYOND

8. Lessons Learned from The Family Dinner Project   139

9. Dinner as a Laboratory for Change   159

10. Extending the Dinner Table to the Wide World   177

   Notes   199

   Resources   213

   Index   217

   About the Author   223

Foreword

I imagine that the readers of this book will come in two flavors: those looking for affirmation and those in need of remediation. The "affirmation" folks—and I can only imagine them because I haven't met many—have picked up this book in order to compare dinnertime parenting notes (and recipes) with Anne Fishel. These people don't have psychic conflicts about food that are left over from childhood. They eat a balanced diet, have control over their work schedules, already cook quite well, never stop at fast-food restaurants, and their children have a sane schedule of after-school activities. Furthermore, Mom and Dad don't answer their cell phones at the table, and there is no sibling taunting at mealtimes. I am filled with admiration for the people in this group. You are amazing (and quite possibly European—maybe even French). You should keep doing what you are doing. No doubt you need support because parenting asks a lot of all mothers and fathers. You will find great comfort in Anne Fishel's delicious writing and her unique combination of experience as a family therapist, mother, and cook.

Then there are the rest of us, the majority of Americans. We need a lot of help in this area. We are not, as Anne explains, ". . . actually having regular family dinners." We cannot get away from work at a predictable hour,

our commutes are too long, or we travel for work and try to stay in touch using Skype or FaceTime. We rush our children from dance lessons to violin recitals to soccer games, grabbing dinner at McDonald's with such frequency that the discarded containers that once held French fries are starting to collect in the back of the car. Or, if we eat at home, we order takeout. One journalist in New York reported that just after he said to his three-year-old son that it was "almost time for dinner," his son disappeared from sight. The dad found him standing at the front door waiting for the delivery person to arrive with the food.

My children are now mostly grown up. One of my biggest regrets about our—my—parenting, is that we did not have more family dinners. I traveled too much, and our daughter played too many sports. And, frankly, my wife and I had complicated feelings about family dinners from the start. My mother was a dreadful cook who yearned to live the high life in New York, meaning that she left my brother and me with maids, who did a terrible job of preparing the unfamiliar recipes Mom left them (and a great job of preparing foods, like chicken jambalaya or fried plantains, from their own countries). My wife's devoutly religious mother turned dinnertime into an occasion for her martyrdom and disappointment in her children. We did not inherit great models of happy dinners. Like most couples, we did the best we could. We averaged one or two family dinners per week. The rest of the time we were on the run—eating in pairs or trios, or grazing while standing at the kitchen counter. We also missed opportunities for collaborative food preparation, which can lead to those unexpected shoulder-to-shoulder conversations with teenagers. Too many memories of our "family dinners" are on vacation or in restaurants and too few at home. We never made the commitment to share stories over our dining room table that I wish we had made.

What would it have taken to get us to try to overcome our family histories and our problematic schedules? If you had asked me five years ago, I would not have known what to say. Now I am clear about my answer: Anne Fishel's book *Home for Dinner*. Dr. Fishel, one of the founders of The Family Dinner Project, has addressed every single issue about family dinners that I have ever encountered in my life or in my therapeutic work with families. Anne takes you by the hand and walks you through whatever minefields you imagine you will encounter in the kitchen. She does it with warmth and humor, with lovely stories about her boys, those food critics who are now young men, and with that amazing husband of hers, who follows her around cleaning up all those pans and utensils.

I offer readers a warning and a confession. Warning: They might wish they were already doing what is outlined in this book. That's okay; not many of us do, but it is never too late. Since reading *Home for Dinner,* my wife and I are determined to cook family dinners for our two granddaughters whenever they come to visit. Our two-year-old granddaughter is already helping to cook: washing vegetables with a brush, whisking the eggs, and stirring the pot.

Finally, my confession: Anne Fishel is both a colleague and a personal friend. I have eaten in her kitchen and in her dining room. She's a phenomenal cook, but more important, she is a gracious hostess. Some of the best dinnertime conversations I have had in the past decade have taken place around her table. She has the ability to make every guest feel welcome, comfortable, and safe. And that's exactly what she does for the readers of this book. I predict that *Home for Dinner* will bring your families closer together.

Michael Thompson, Ph.D.,
clinical psychologist and
New York Times bestselling coauthor of
*Raising Cain: Protecting the
Emotional Life of Boys*

Acknowledgments

When it came to writing this book, I've been so grateful to have had "many cooks in the kitchen."

My heartfelt and enduring thanks to my friends and colleagues at The Family Dinner Project, an inspiring, creative, and talented group, who have taught me so much over the past few years. I have enlisted several team members to read chapters of this book in manuscript, and their input has greatly improved the book: Shelly London, Ashley Sandvi, Lynn Barendsen, Wendy Fischman, and Amy Yelin. Other FDP members have contributed to this book in many other ways: Bob Stains, Jono Reduker, John Sarrouf, Grace Taylor, Paromita De, Allissa Wickham, and Bri DeRosa. A special thanks to Shelly London, whose support of my work with FDP, and of my writing in particular, has meant the world to me.

Several others have lent their time and expertise to reading chapters and providing me with invaluable suggestions and feedback: Tai Katzenstein, Laura Weisberg, and Carol DeCouto.

Some of the ideas in this book have gotten first passes in other forums. I am grateful to David Rubin for inviting me to give a grand rounds at Cornell Medical School many years ago, when I was just beginning to formulate my ideas about family dinners. I was glad to be invited by the Mayo

Clinic to present on this topic with Bob Stains at the Transform Conference in 2013. Several sections have appeared as blog posts on NPR's now defunct Public Radio Kitchen—thanks to Sue McCrory for asking me to be part of that. Thanks to Tristan Gorrindo, my good friend, for inviting me to write about family dinners for the Massachusetts General Hospital Clay Center. Thanks, too, to Julie Silver for her early interest in this project.

I am fortunate to be part of a writers' group at MGH that has provided me with support and good humor during our early Friday morning meetings. My fellow writers have given me essential feedback about this book's tone and attitude: Laura Prager, Tia Horner, Lisa Solomon, Linda Forsythe, Cindy Moore, and Bob Reifsnyder.

Over the past many decades, a group of fellow mental health professionals—"The Ladies," as my sons dubbed them—have had my back for professional and personal issues, great and small: Paula Rauch, Nancy Bridges, Beth Harrington, Chris McElroy, and Sue Wolff. And with this book, they were always ready to buoy me up or troubleshoot, as well as try out recipes for the book.

I am grateful to many families—both in my practice and whom I've met at community dinners in Cambridge, Lynn, and Revere, Massachusetts, as well as in West Concord, Minnesota. In addition, the child psychiatry fellows at MGH, from 2002 to the present, have kept me on my toes and helped me fine-tune my clinical use of family dinners.

Other friends have helped nourish me with food and conversation (and often conversation about food), and I particularly thank Nancy Gardiner, Franny Taliaferro, Ginger Chappell, Eva Schoenfeld, Linette Liebling, Carolyn Wong, and Marti Straus.

Along the way several people were willing to let me learn from them about their expertise regarding food, families, cooking, nutrition, or gardening: I am indebted to David Gass, Tristram Stuart, Carly Zimmerman, Caryn Roth, Jillian Katz, Geoff Lukas, Lisa Price, Mai Uchida, Beverly Woo, Carol Singer, Ellen O'Donnell, Susan Swick, and Patricia Papernow.

I feel so honored by Michael Thompson's response to this book. His wise and deep work on boys has been a guide to me as a mother.

I am so appreciative of the hardworking, dedicated AMACOM team. Thanks to each of them for their expert contributions to this book: Irene

Majuk, Jenny Wesselmann, Rosemary Carlough, Therese Mausser, Cathleen Ouderkirk, and Erika Spelman. I especially want to thank my editor at AMACOM, Ellen Kadin, whose support and wise judgment, from soup to nuts, has been so important. And my agent, Linda Konner, whose belief in this book from the beginning and her availability along the way for sensible feedback have helped sustain me.

I am additionally grateful for the editorial help graciously given by Ginny Carroll and Carol Boker. And, to Louis Greenstein, a big thanks for his firm but kind editorial handling of the final manuscript.

Most of all, I want to thank my family. My parents taught me the importance of family dinners, and they live on in me and my family. My mother, Edith Fishel, was my model for the virtues of speedy cooking. She wanted to get out of the kitchen and join in the dinner conversation as quickly as possible. My father, James Fishel, was simply the best dinnertime storyteller I've ever known. And I have such gratitude for my sister, Elizabeth Fishel—a superb writer, cook, and parent. Not only did she enliven our childhood table with her incomparable wit, she has shared her recipes and parenting tips with me as a fellow mother of sons. More than once, she joined me and my son Joe for cooking classes, and she always made them memorable and joyful occasions. Her thoughtful, astute feedback on several chapters is also much appreciated.

I am most indebted to my sons and my husband. Gabe and Joe have been my staunchest supporters and my most honest critics when it comes to cooking. I have learned much from them about how to cook with care and not just with speed. Nothing is more fun than cooking with them and then lingering at the table. They make every dinner a special event. And to my husband, Chris, who offers his unstinting support in the kitchen and everywhere else. I cannot begin to express my appreciation for his unwavering encouragement, good cheer, and willingness to drop whatever he was doing to read each chapter as soon as I was done. Most of all, I treasure his companionship, his love, and the way that he makes me feel at home, whether it's dinnertime or not.

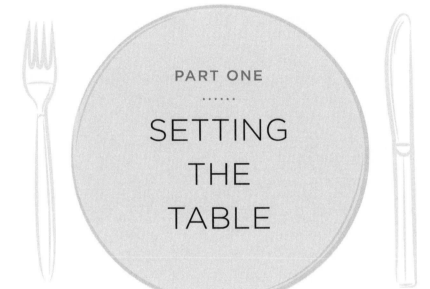

PART ONE

......

SETTING
THE
TABLE

1

Welcome to the Table

Experiences with food have played a central role in my life as a wife, mother, teacher, therapist, and community organizer, and they constitute the raw ingredients for this book.

I first made a commitment to cooking tasty family dinners twenty-two years ago when my husband gave up smoking after our second son was born. It seemed like a fair trade—one oral pleasure to nourish and delight him in exchange for another that could kill him. In the bargain, I soon realized I had stumbled onto something with unexpected benefits for everyone in my family. Some nights, my two young sons wanted to help—at first just banging pots around but later stirring the soup, washing the greens, and pulling basil leaves off their stems. Their kitchen participation turned them into stakeholders at dinner—they wanted to try their own handiwork. Other nights, they preferred to play with their father. On those nights, I was left alone in the kitchen, and cooking became the one quiet, meditative time of my day. It felt like a guilty pleasure. In the guise of being a good mother, I earned some time to myself.

We ate dinner in the kitchen around a wooden table. It was cozy when our sons were young, but it became pleasantly cramped as they stretched out to more than six feet tall. My sons were adventurous and demanding eaters. They egged me on to try a new dish almost every night despite my wish to build up a repertoire of recipes that I could make in my sleep (a state I hovered close to as a working mother with two young kids).

While I wasn't exactly Julie Powell trying all of Julia Child's recipes, I did try to keep up with my sons' curiosity about new foods, and I experimented with dishes I'd never eaten before. Once, we spent an entire afternoon trying to open a coconut they'd spied at the supermarket after seeing one in a Babar the Elephant book. The coconut remained stubbornly shut despite my assaults on it with hammer, screwdriver, and knife. Finally, I cleared out the street below and we threw it out a third-floor window. This was effective, but it meant that we couldn't use the coconut milk, which supposedly was the best part.

Another time, we made limeade by squeezing about twenty limes like mad. Days later, my older son, the chief squeezer, developed a mysterious rash in a C-shape around his thumb and index finger. After consultations with numerous pediatricians who were stumped, a nurse diagnosed it as a rash that develops when sun interacts with lime juice. Other mishaps occurred from time to time when I tried a new recipe. I recall a hollandaise sauce that tasted like papier-mâché. But I like to think that my sons and I learned to appreciate one another's willingness to try new things even when the results were inedible and never to be repeated.

As my sons got older, they began to cook dishes and then courses and then whole meals on their own. One night a few years ago, I came home from seeing patients at Massachusetts General Hospital, feeling tired and depleted. As I entered the house, I was struck by the homey smell of melting cheese and saw that the kitchen was strewn with cookbooks. Knowing I would be home late, my younger son, Joe, had driven to the store and purchased ingredients to make dinner. And not just any dinner, but a blue cheese soufflé accompanied by a salad of beets, spinach, and roasted walnuts. He was headed off to college in a few months, and I knew he'd learned one important lesson at home: the power of a home-cooked meal to bring cheer at the end of a long day.

Now that my sons live in their own apartments, I am proud that they are competent and creative cooks. (My husband is another issue, but I didn't raise him!) My older son, Gabe, can throw a dinner party for a dozen friends, with stuffed eggplant, butterflied chicken, and a risotto made with from-scratch chicken stock. Joe makes dinner in a shoebox-size New York kitchen and then takes leftovers to work for lunch.

But I don't want to leave you with the impression that my family dinners have been a seamless affair with everyone praising my culinary efforts, asking to chop the onions, and offering to wash the dishes. Making dinner night after night was sometimes tedious and frustrating. I often felt too tired to cook, or didn't have the ingredients I needed, or had started cooking so late that the kids had spoiled their appetites on snacks by the time dinner was ready, or I couldn't think of a menu that would please everyone, or I threw up my hands when the kids' rehearsals and athletic practices were scheduled at the dinner hour.

Home for Dinner is intended for any parent who feels similarly frustrated, bored, or overwhelmed by the prospect of making dinner night after night. Think of this book as a well-stocked pantry that has sauces to perk up a tired meal or a can of beans to add nutrition to a familiar dish. Perhaps, one night when you've run out of ideas of what to cook for dinner or what to talk about at the table, you'll remember something you read here and pull it out, like grabbing something from a back shelf. My hope is that you can dip into it tonight, next week, or next year for something to make dinner easier or more enjoyable. There's nothing here that is meant to be a heavy lift, nothing that requires an overhaul of what you're already doing.

With all this talk of home-cooked meals, I'd be remiss without making the following confession: My favorite family dinner of the week was the one I didn't cook. Every Friday night, I used to take a nap. While I slept, my husband and sons would order takeout—either oversize tubs of pasta that fed us all weekend or greasy eggrolls and lo mein. I didn't care that the food wasn't particularly good or nutritious. I was just grateful for that delicious nap!

My family dinners weren't just tiring to make; several years ago, they also became quite contentious. When my sons were young teens, they briefly turned into restaurant critics who analyzed each meal I made within an inch of its life. Finally, I did something I'm not a bit proud of: I went on strike, refusing to cook another meal until they changed their tune and showed some appreciation for my efforts. My husband crossed the picket line to cook for them, but out of loyalty to me, he didn't try too hard. After a few days, they urged me to reconsider my position, and we hammered out a new agreement: My sons would offer constructive and brief criticism about any new dish I prepared and would decide whether it was worthy of being made a second time; however, they would not bad-mouth any meal that had already been given their stamp of approval. More significantly, Joe, then thirteen, would start making meat dishes for his brother and father, a marked change from the fish and chicken menus that I'd been preparing.

This sharing of the kitchen with my omnivore son took me full circle: As a teenager, I'd renounced meat and demanded that my beef-and-burger cooking mother share her kitchen with me so that I could make vegetarian meals. I was familiar with the ways that food choices can provide an outlet to redefine the roles between a parent and an adolescent, and now it was my turn. Family dinner can be an everyday laboratory for experimenting with new roles and behaviors. (You'll find more on this in Chapter 9.)

At the same time that I was exploring the pleasures of my own family dinners, I was also developing an interest in food in my work as a psychologist. As a young therapist I'd worked with women who had eating disorders, and I saw how these vulnerable patients had developed conflicted relationships with food. Some would cook elaborate meals for their families but rarely sat down to eat with them. I wasn't surprised when, years later, I read in the scientific literature that girls who don't have family dinners are more likely to develop eating disorders.

My home office is in the basement of our house, just beneath the kitchen. Many nights I used to pop a chicken or lasagna in the oven just before seeing a family for a late-afternoon session. One night as the unmistakable aroma of roast chicken wafted through the heating vents, I remember feeling a bit guilty when I checked the clock to see how soon until dinner. A teenager in the family half-jokingly asked if they could stay for dinner. I had an epiphany right then. Knowing what I did about all the benefits of nightly family dinners, I wanted to say to this family, "Your hour would be better spent making dinner together, eating it, and talking around the table rather than sitting in my office. Here are some cookbooks—now go!" I kept this private reverie to myself, but from then on, I found a way to ask every family I saw in therapy whether they have dinner together and, if not, what might be getting in their way.

As a family therapist for more than twenty-five years, I've developed a belief that helping families develop new dinner rituals can be a form of healing. I have tried to help many families reconnect by developing a nightly commitment to having dinner together. In some families the new roles created around cooking, choosing menus, and picking topics for dinner conversation have been transformative. (I share some of these stories in Chapter 9.)

At Massachusetts General Hospital, I also train child and adult psychiatry residents and child psychology interns how to be family therapists. There is no more powerful class than the one where I ask students to interview each other about the family dinners they experienced while growing up. In those few minutes, students "get" the major principles of family systems theory, and they learn about each other in ways that are unguarded and unrehearsed. It's so much easier to talk about your dinnertime than about your sex life or the role you play in your family.

Similarly, in Chapter 8, I'll ask you to think about your own dinnertime—both the one that you have with your current family and the one that you had with the family you grew up with. Perhaps you'll want to change some parts of your current dinner ritual. These changes can provide a powerful way to bring your family closer, to ask a child to assume a new responsibility, or to create more lively, interesting conversations—changes that you can develop in a playful, nonintrusive way and without going to therapy.

Most of us know intuitively that family dinners are good for families. Dramatic research findings show that family dinners can also inoculate us against a host of ills, from substance abuse and obesity to low achievement scores and behavioral problems. Studies show that dinner conversation is an even more potent vocabulary-booster for our children than reading aloud to them. Other studies show that the stories we tell around the kitchen table help our children to build resilience and self-esteem. (I'll summarize the scientific literature for you in Chapter 2.) What else can families do that takes only an hour a day and packs such a punch?

Food is to families what sex is to couples, what a sandbox is to children, or what music is to adolescents. It's a medium of play—a way for families to have pleasure with one another while expressing their values, roles, hopes, and identities. Most of the families I see in my psychotherapy practice want to improve communication, strengthen ties, and promote the well-being of their children. While an hour of weekly family therapy can be helpful, a nightly commitment to family dinners can be transformative. Of course, food isn't a family's only means of self-expression, just as music isn't the lifeblood of all adolescents. Many happy families surely get meals over as quickly as possible or get takeout every night. But what else do families do three times a day, seven times a week? When you compare food to sex (which a couple has to do only once to make a family), you get some idea of its centrality.

But the power of nightly dinners comes from more than the food. It's an excuse to bring your family together. It can even offer the starting point for conversation, since families tend to spend about one-fifth of their table talk focused on the food—"Please pass the salt," or "This meat is overdone," or "How did you cook the carrots? They're delicious."

The real power of family dinners comes from the particular quality of conversation around the dinner table. Unlike talk we have during carpool or while tucking in a child at bedtime, conversation at the dinner table is likely to be linguistically complex, cognitively challenging, and very engaging. Dinner conversation, rich in nutrients, is a place to seed important values. I have noticed that the conversations I try to promote in family therapy are just the kind that can naturally occur around the dinner table. In therapy and at the table, family members are encouraged to speak about their own experience while being listened to with curiosity and emotional attunement. The family comes away from both experiences with the sense that being together is more than the sum of its individual parts. What is created is something greater—the sense of belonging to a family that has its own set of stories and identities.

What I hear from my patients, however, is that they often don't know how to talk to their children once they have them gathered around the table. So in this book I provide you with tools you can use in the dinner hour to have conversations that develop resilience, encourage empathy, build connection, promote individuality, and help make your children moral citizens. The dinner hour is an ideal time and place to seed and incubate these conversations, which can then be carried on during other times of the day. (In Chapter 6, I translate for you the insights I've learned as a family therapist to conversations that your family can have around the dinner table.)

Until about three years ago, I thought I knew everything I needed to about family dinners. I was conversant with the scientific literature, which demonstrated the connection between regular family dinners and benefits to the mind, body, and spirit of individual members. Of course, I was sold on family dinners even before I knew about the research because of the fun I had with my own family around our kitchen table. I routinely asked families I saw in therapy about their dinners and had figured out ways to help them make changes at dinner that fanned out across the day. In my teaching role, I thought I'd even been able to convince some of the next generation of family therapists to respect the power of family dinners. So I wasn't prepared for the transformation in my thinking and practice after I received an email from Shelly London, a retired senior corporate executive who was a fellow at Harvard working on developing projects to promote ethical thinking. At a lunch that stretched over hours, we discussed the importance of family dinner in a culture where families are starved for time to spend with one another. She was excited to think about family dinner, the one time of the day when families still congregate, as a time and place to promote meaningful conversation.

Shelly assembled a disparate group of kindred spirits—a chef, a web designer, a therapist, educators, researchers, and community activists—who were committed to all the ways that dinners are nourishing to families. After many conversations with each other and with families, we developed resources to help families with all the elements they would need for a satisfying dinner—quick and healthy recipes, interesting conversation starters, and games to encourage kids to stay longer at the table. We tried out these resources on pilot families, interviewing them before and after a kick-off community dinner to find out what worked and what didn't. And we formed a growing grassroots organization, The Family Dinner Project, which provides families and communities with the online and in-person resources to promote healthy food, fun, and conversation about things that matter.

While I knew a lot about why family dinner is important, my work at
The Family Dinner Project has helped hone my ability to translate the
"why" into the "how." Through working with many communities in person and with individual families online, we've discovered ways to help
families make the changes they want, with tools we've gathered from many
different worlds—culinary, therapeutic, and educational—and from innovative families across the country.

Not only that. In this work, my definition of family has expanded beyond the traditional nuclear family. Now I think of family as any group
that feels like home: a neighborhood that gathers around a backyard clay
oven to make pizzas, a gathering of friends at college, young adults living
with friends who are part of their chosen family, or a community dinner at
a school, church hall, or diner. I no longer just think about helping one
family at a time, as I do in my therapy practice. Instead, at The Family
Dinner Project we hope that the benefits of family dinners will spread as
part of the cultural discourse, much as "Fasten your seat belt" and "No
smoking" have.

With The Family Dinner Project, I have worked with communities of
families in low-income urban neighborhoods, such as Lynn, Massachusetts,
and with rural families like those in Dodge County, Minnesota. My colleagues and I have helped families set their own goals for changing family
dinners—from wanting to have more enjoyment at dinner, to eating more
nutritious food, to having more meaningful conversation, to fighting less,
to getting more help with the cooking and cleaning up. With our team at
The Family Dinner Project I have offered families tools and resources to
make those changes. Moreover, I have seen how these ideas have grabbed
hold and spread from family to family. This is not the family dinner of the
1950s, where a mother is toiling away by herself in the kitchen and waiting
for her husband, the sole provider, to arrive home for dinner every night
at 6 p.m. (The insights from The Family Dinner Project are discussed in
Chapter 8.)

Although most families endorse the idea of family dinners, surveys of
American families indicate that most parents are not actually having regular family dinners. As a family therapist and a community activist, I have
learned a lot about what families need in order to make change happen.

Families need to make a commitment to setting aside time for dinners. They need help to keep food preparation simple and to find ways to involve multiple family members; they need games and playful strategies at the table to make it fun; and they need inspiration to make dinnertime feel like a meaningful ritual.

While the scientific research about dinnertime is compelling, I know that it is not enough all by itself to bring families to the dinner table. In this book you will also learn how to implement a nightly dinner with tips on how to involve kids of all ages in cooking, how to make the dinner table conversation enjoyable and stimulating, and how to rotate food choices and roles so that dinner is a lively and interesting occasion, rather than a chore to be gotten through night after night. I also share about forty kid-tested, favorite dinner recipes from all over the world, most of which can be made in about thirty minutes.

Home for Dinner is an invitation back to the table, with a little science to explain the mental health and intellectual benefits of regular dinner, with tips to tailor mealtime to children of different ages (Chapter 3), with stories and recipes from other families (Chapters 4 and 8), and with many ideas to make dinner a source of play for all family members (Chapters 5, 6, and 7). I'll also suggest ways that family dinner can spur kids and families to social activism in the wider world (Chapter 10).

If time is the obstacle to creating nightly dinners, you may want to think again. If you are helping to head a household, nightly dinners are high-impact: You get to nourish your family, prevent a host of problems, increase your children's cognitive abilities, and provide pleasure and delight that they can build on for the rest of their lives. You can also use dinner as a time for your children to explore their connections to families from different cultures, and to their place in the web of living things.

The table is set. Come join the conversation.

2

What's So Great About Family Dinners?
What the Research Can Tell Us

Over the last two decades, many scientific studies have confirmed what you have known intuitively for a long time: Sitting down to a family meal is good for the brain, the spirit, and the health of all family members.[1]

Recent studies link frequent family dinners with a host of teenage behaviors that parents pray for: lower rates of substance abuse, pregnancy, and depression, as well as higher grade-point averages and self-esteem.[2] Other research has found that dinners are more powerful than reading aloud in building literacy in young children. Family dinners have even been shown to disrupt the cycle of alcoholism from one generation to the next.[3] The icing on the cake? Regular family meals have been shown to lower obesity rates among children.

Perhaps the heft of the research will be enough to convince you to try some new strategies to bring your kids to the table a few more times a week, or to linger a while longer. Sometimes scientific data can motivate us to change behavior. For example, I always knew that exercise was good for me, but when I read in a scientific journal that it was as good as taking antidepressant medication, I felt even more motivated to hop on my elliptical machine, even when a nap seemed so much more appealing. The scientific confirmation of what I knew in my heart transformed my knowledge into action. I hope the evidence I'm offering here will have the same effect.

———

The science concerning family meals falls into three broad categories: Evidence shows that family dinners enhance children's intellectual functioning, promote mental health, and improve physical health and nutrition.[4] All of the studies use five meals a week as the minimum number necessary to have an effect, but this figure may be arbitrary, and there are inconsistencies in how researchers arrive at this "magic number." Some researchers include breakfasts, along with dinners, to get to the number five. Others compare families who eat five or more with those who eat less than two to see effects, but don't examine whether three or four nightly dinners are sufficient. But the emphasis on the number of dinners per week skirts the influence of the *quality* of the mealtime experience, which may be a more powerful factor than the *quantity* of meals.

I don't think any researcher has made a case for dinner being more powerful than breakfast or lunch. In industrialized societies, however, dinner tends to be the meal that families are most likely to eat together. (In agrarian communities, families may also gather for a big lunch in the middle of the day.) In twenty-first-century America, breakfast tends to be eaten on the run as kids scramble to catch their school buses and parents battle rush hour to get to work. So, while I don't think there is anything inherently special about dinner, the fact is, it's the meal most likely to be attended by your whole family and eaten in a leisurely way.

Many, though not all of the studies, come with a caveat: It might not be the meal itself that makes the difference. That is, it's possible that children who eat a lot of family meals together also have more supervision, more structure, and less time to get into trouble. Or perhaps families who dine together also read and take more walks together. In other words, the beneficial effects we attribute to family dinners might actually be part of something broader, such as being in a very connected and organized family. Some studies do control for these variables and still find that family meals create unique and positive outcomes that cannot be attributed to any other cause.

Several studies could be criticized for saying they are measuring the effects of nightly family dinners when really they are measuring the effects of a family's ability to supervise, organize, and value intimacy. However, I don't think it matters. Why? It seems likely that having family dinners develops these family strengths. Families who have a nightly dinner become more organized and more connected. I'm reminded of the old adage "fake it until you make it." If exercise will make you less depressed, but you have to be less depressed before you can start exercising, you might be told to fake it at first. Try to get yourself exercising so you will begin to reap the benefits. Similarly, a family that is disconnected and disorganized can focus on family dinners, and in the process become more connected and organized.

Recent articles have suggested that the benefits of family dinners are only as powerful as the quality of the relationships around the table.[5] If family members sit in stony silence, if parents yell at each other or scold their kids, dinner won't confer positive benefits. Teens with poor relationships with parents *away* from the dinner table do not derive as many benefits from dining with their parents as teens who have strong relationships with their parents. But that's a chicken-and-egg issue, since dinner remains one of the most predictable times of the day when relationships among family members can be strengthened. Sharing a pork shoulder won't magically transform a difficult parent–child relationship, but avoiding the communication opportunities that dinner provides certainly won't improve it. Rather, dinner may be the one time of the day when a parent and a child enjoy something positive together—a well-cooked roast or a joke—and then, that small moment can build on moments away from the table.

FAMILY DINNERS ARE GOOD FOR THE BRAIN, THE SPIRIT, AND THE BODY

I have organized this chapter so that you can look at the intellectual, psychological, and physical benefits of family dinners, and within each category, you can pay special attention to different age groups, specifically young children (under age six); school-age children (ages six to twelve); and teens (ages twelve to eighteen). Later in this chapter I offer some research-based answers to the question of why there are so many benefits to family dinners.

Intellectual benefits for kids under age six

Over the past thirty years, researchers at the Harvard School of Education have found consistently that, as a way to boost children's vocabulary, talking to them during dinner is even better than reading to them. And children with well-developed vocabularies will have an easier time learning to read, since they won't have to decode the meaning and sound out the word at the same time. Good readers not only understand the meaning of stories, but they also bring knowledge of the world to their reading, and they have big vocabularies—all skills that can be learned at the dinner table.

Harvard researchers have also found that dinner table conversations are different from other family conversations.[6] Unlike talk we have in the car or while walking a child to school, conversation at the dinner table is likely to include new vocabulary, storytelling, and a high degree of engagement. That's because when families eat together, parents expect that the kids will sit and talk for more than a few minutes. Conversation often focuses on a single topic, with input from several members and with multiple comments that are often complex. Dinner conversation is ideal for incubating your children's language development.

Two types of mealtime talk are particularly potent: explanatory talk and narrative talk. Explanatory talk is often initiated by a child's questions (for example, "Daddy, why doesn't everyone have the same amount of money as everyone else?") or by a parent stopping the conversation to make sure that a child understands what is being discussed (for example, "Why do you think some people live on the streets instead of in houses?"). Narrative talk includes the stories that each member tells about the day, as well as conversation about past events in the family and plans for the future. In many families, each child is asked to tell about his or her day, and as children grow up, they are expected to tell more complex stories. Stories have the potential to teach important family values, to entertain, and to stretch a child's understanding of the world.

One recent study analyzed 160 mealtime conversations of children age three to five to try to figure out what kinds of conversation improved vocabulary and reading skills.[7] Explanatory talk and narrative talk each accounted for about 15 percent of mealtime conversation. (The other

70 percent was taken up with talk about food and by parental commands to behave. For example, "These string beans are too mushy" and "Don't talk while chewing.") They found that both explanatory and narrative dinner conversation help language development in ways that show up years later. For example, children who participated in more narrative talk at age three had higher reading achievement scores at age seven. And it had even more far-reaching benefits: Children who engaged in a lot of narrative talk at age five had a greater understanding of words at age eleven. Engaging in explanatory talk also reaped fruitful results later on: Three-year-olds who engaged in explanatory talk had higher reading and higher vocabulary scores four years later.

These researchers also counted the number of "rare words" that the kids used. Rare words are defined as those not found on a list of the 3,000 most common words. The researchers tallied 2,000 rare words, and it turned out only 143 came from parents reading to their children. The real jackpot for rare words came from the dinner table, where 1,000 were learned. This exposure to a large vocabulary is one of the most powerful predictors of reading abilities. As Catherine Snow, one of the principal researchers explains, "The frequency at which they (the children) were exposed to rare words at (age) three and four predicted their kindergarten vocabulary. We found vocabulary at kindergarten was a very good predictor of reading comprehension throughout the rest of their lives." In Chapter 6, I offer ways parents can include this kind of powerful talk at the dinner table.

Intellectual benefits for school-age kids

The intellectual benefits of regular dinnertime don't stop at preschool. Studies have found that children who have regular dinners perform better academically in elementary school. Researchers found that regular mealtime was an even more powerful predictor of higher achievement scores than time spent in school, doing homework, playing sports, or doing art.[8] In fact, kids of all ages, both male and female, growing up in poor or wealthy families, and regardless of race or ethnicity, reaped academic benefits by having regular family dinners.

In another study, a researcher followed families from the time the kids were in preschool until they were in early elementary school.[9] She found that when parents were strongly committed to organizing family dinners when kids were young, and when they valued the emotional connections they felt during mealtime, their kids experienced benefits when they were older. Specifically, children who participated in family dinners at age four scored higher on tests of academic achievement years later. Similar results were found in a study of boys raised in low-income, single-parent African-American families.[10] When mealtime rituals were regular and predictable, elementary-age boys did better at school. The authors hypothesized that the routines at home provided the boys with a sense of control, which helped reduce the likelihood of developing behavior problems.

Academic benefits for adolescents, too

Researchers at Columbia University's National Center on Addiction and Substance Abuse (CASA) have reported a consistent association, over several years, between family dinner frequency and teen academic performance. According to CASA, adolescents who ate family dinners five to seven times a week were twice as likely to get A's in school as those who ate dinner with their families fewer than three times a week.[11]

FAMILY DINNER IS GOOD FOR MENTAL HEALTH

When it comes to the mental health benefits of family dinners, researchers seem most interested in their impact on teens. This weighting of research may reflect the increase in risky behaviors that adolescents engage in, and so researchers take an interest in such activities as family dinners that can protect adolescents. A pile of studies have found a correlation between regular family dinners and the reduction of high-risk behaviors like smoking, binge drinking, marijuana use, violence, school problems, and sexual activity.[12] This connection was more important than church attendance or good grades in predicting lack of drug and alcohol use and teenage pregnancy. In a large study of more than 5,000 adolescents in Minnesota, the researchers concluded that regular family dinners were associated with lower rates of depression and suicidal thoughts, as well as higher self-esteem. They also found a decrease in substance abuse, which they attributed to the way that teens who dine with their families regularly are more closely supervised and monitored.[13] Even more intriguing, these same researchers reported that girls who participated in frequent family dinners as early teens grew up to have less substance abuse five years later.[14]

In addition, several researchers have found that girls who eat regularly with their families are less likely to develop eating disorders. In one study, when girls ate five or more meals a week with their parents, the risk of developing an eating disorder was lowered by thirty percent.[15] And these findings were similar when an ethnically diverse group of 5,000 adolescents was surveyed. Those who ate regular family dinners experienced less chronic dieting and less binge eating.[16] Family dinners have been shown to reduce problems at school and are even associated with teens having more of a sense of purpose and a more positive view of the future than their peers.[17]

PHYSICAL HEALTH BENEFITS

The research also shows profound physical health benefits in terms of weight control, better nutritional intake, and teaching good eating habits.

Benefits for young children

In one study, researchers found that kindergartners who watched more TV and ate fewer family meals were more likely to be overweight by the time they were in third grade.[18] Put another way, combining early good-eating habits with turning off the TV will pay off years later. Regular family dinners prevent grazing between meals and allow kids to learn to pay attention to cues of fullness when TV isn't distracting them.

Benefits for school-age kids

In a study of school-age children, those who had more regular meals with their parents had more healthful dietary patterns, including eating more fruits and vegetables, fewer fried foods and soft drinks, and more vitamins and micronutrients.[19]

But, it isn't just the presence of healthy foods that leads to less obesity. Researchers also discovered a connection between the atmosphere at the table and obesity rates: A parenting style that is controlling and restrictive toward food was associated with higher rates of obesity in children.[20] According to another study, parents who didn't show genuine concern for their children and were disengaged during mealtime were more likely to have overweight children.[21]

Some studies show a connection between regular family dinners and the reduction of symptoms in some medical disorders, such as asthma.[22] Children who ate regular family dinners had lower levels of anxiety, a symptom linked with asthma. Children with asthma have a lot to feel anxious about, like missing school or having to rush to an emergency room or having to remember to use a mechanical ventilator. Family dinners provide a prime time to observe a child's symptoms and check in about whether he has been taking his medication.[23]

Benefits for adolescents

Teens who dine with their parents consume more fruits and vegetables, as well as fewer fried foods and soft drinks, and they are less likely to be overweight.[24] These results were replicated among low-income and single-parent families. And these same kids will continue to eat healthy meals once they are on their own as young adults.[25] So family dinners are an investment in the future health of your children.

WHY DOES FAMILY DINNER HAVE SUCH POWERFUL EFFECTS?

If, as a family, we farmed together each morning, rehearsed in a string quartet every afternoon, or stitched quilts on the porch in the evening, we would stay connected. But in today's culture, having dinner as a family is the most doable way to hang out together; there are few other settings where the family gathers.

Dinner is a family's prime time to connect

Mealtimes are one of the few opportunities during the day when parents can influence their children's behavior and development. Families who eat together most nights of the week know what is going on in one another's lives; they feel connected. When teenagers were asked when, other than dinner, they talked to their parents, most said that it was in the car, an opportunity that isn't always available in urban settings and dries up when kids start driving themselves.[26]

Kids who eat dinner with their parents experience less stress. They feel as if their parents really know them and that they have a better relationship with them.[27] Dinner is an opportunity, a container, and a canvas. How families use that opportunity, fill its contents, and paint on it can be changed, amplified, and made more enjoyable. There is nothing inherently magical about dinner, but for most families it is simply the most reliable time of the day to connect with one another. It is this connection that provides a powerful seat belt on the potholed road of childhood and adolescence.

Perhaps the presence of food adds a sensory pleasure that softens the context in which parents may probe their children for information about the day. Hungry kids are usually sullen and irritable; children who are enjoying a meal may feel much more relaxed and willing to talk.

Family dinners lead to better nutrition

Compared to the nutritional value of eating in restaurants, family dinners are significantly lower in calories and saturated fat.[28] This is particularly true when family dinners are compared to fast-food meals, with their oversize portions and uninhibited dosing of sugar, salt, and fat. People tend to eat more fruits and vegetables at home than in restaurants. When parents eat with their teens, they can model and monitor what their kids are eating. Most adults aren't going to start dinner with ice cream or make a meal that consists of only a bowl of pasta with butter.

When families sit down together at home, their portions tend to be smaller. Also, when kids eat at the table with their families, they may eat more slowly than they would if wolfing down a meal in front of a computer or TV. This slower pace, brought about by conversation, allows the brain to register cues that tell a person he has had enough food to satisfy his hunger.

Dinner as a ritual conveys meaning and stability

If we define "rituals" as repeated actions with symbolic meaning that are enacted at a particular time and place, then we can agree that neither ministers, imams, nor rabbis have a lock on them. In fact, family therapists have been touting rituals for decades. Rituals range from occasional, formal observances, such as communions, weddings, and funerals, to everyday, highly choreographed activities, such as reading three picture books, singing a folk song, and kissing your child goodnight.

Family dinner is the quintessential ritual.[29] It has a prescribed use of time and space, which sets the experience off from usual activities. It typically occurs at roughly the same time, say 6 p.m., and in the same place, a dining room or kitchen. One of the most important features of a ritual is that it has a protected boundary of time around it so that families need to know when it will begin and about how long it will take to unfold.

Another important feature of a ritual is that it can be both scripted and unscripted. The scripted parts of dinner are ones that we do over and over so we don't have to reinvent the experience each time. In most families, for example, everyone sits in the same seat each night. My sons liked to sit on the cushioned banquette, while my husband and I sat in seats that allowed us to spring up from the table to fetch more food and water. Other scripted aspects include the way that I always served the food and my husband always washed the dishes. These were the lines in which the dinner got painted.

The unscripted parts of dinner are up for grabs each night. They make mealtime interesting and a vital part of the day. After all, if every aspect of dinner is routine and predictable, the juice gets squeezed out of the ritual. Adding a new dish, trying out a new conversation starter, eating the dinner in a different part of the house, sitting in different seats, or occasionally inviting guests can encourage flexibility.

Dinner, like other rituals, has symbols that lend meaning and emotion. Food is the predominant symbol, and it can be imbued with meanings about care, nurture, and love, or about power and control, or about adventure and the exploration of new tastes. Because of the meaning a family gives to food, family members know the difference between a home-cooked meal and takeout.

Rituals help create a shared family identity and a sense of belonging. As one mother offered when asked about the importance of dinner: "Sitting down to dinner is like coming together to make a whole, like pieces of a puzzle." This sense of the whole being greater than the sum of its parts and everyone belonging to the whole is an important aspect of the dinner ritual.

Rituals also connect us to previous generations, as when we cook foods for our children that our parents made for us or cook foods that belong to a country from which we emigrated. Our parents and grandparents live on in us and in our children by what we eat and the stories we tell. One researcher observed that rituals are like "condensed, prepackaged training modules intended to convey to all family members the important facts about family identity."[30]

When rituals remind us of our cultural heritage and ties to a wider family, they can help create a family identity that is bigger than our immediate family. But some parents may deliberately choose to avoid repeating the rituals that they grew up with because they were joyless, hollow, haphazard, or controlling. While rituals can offer continuity to previous generations, they can also be used to mark a discontinuity, an intention to organize family life differently than one's parents did. A dinner ritual can create a fresh start and a way to interrupt earlier family patterns.

By occurring during a time and place set off from the daily fray of individual pursuits, rituals can allow a greater expression of feelings. This is akin to therapy, which also has a boundary around it by taking place in an office at a scheduled time. At both dinner and therapy, a boundary allows individuals to feel freer to explore and express themselves, in part, because there is an ending to it, and because it is set apart from daily life, so the usual conventions of conversation are suspended.

Ang Lee, the director of the film *Eat Drink Man Woman*, explains the role of ritual in his tale about a Korean family who congregate every Sunday for an emotionally charged dinner: "Sometimes the things children need to hear most are often the things that parents find hardest to say, and vice versa. When that happens, we resort to ritual."[31]

Perhaps most important, rituals, in their repetitive predictability, offer stability. There is something very comforting about knowing that one part of your day is going to unfold in pretty much the same way, day after day. Rituals punctuate a world that often feels frenzied and out of control, and these semi-choreographed events are as welcome to adults as to children. The structure also allows for spontaneity, the way that knowing the tune to a song allows a saxophonist to let loose with improvisation.

If kids are eating dinner, what are they not doing?

When kids are home for dinner, it means they *aren't* roaming the streets and getting into trouble. Home for dinner means that your kids are spending some time away from the computer. I don't know of any studies that look at this factor, but I think it may be significant. Having dinner is a social behavior that may knock out some other, less healthy, behaviors.

3

One Size Dinner
Doesn't Fit All Ages

Y ou wouldn't expect your sixteen-year-old daughter to keep wearing the one-piece footed "bunny suits" of her preschool years. So why would you assume that your child's involvement in family dinner will remain unchanged over the course of growing up? When it goes well, the family dinner transforms along with your kids. Your child's appetite, ability to cook, and readiness to participate in dinner conversation all change dramatically from infancy through young adulthood. A dinner plan for toddlers that involves finger foods and a modest expectation for time spent sitting at the table will look very different for your adolescent children who can discuss a broad range of topics but who need different enticements to keep nightly dinners on their busy dance cards.

Understanding the changing challenges of dinnertime and seeing them in terms of the developmental changes that occur as your children continue to grow allows you to shape dinner to bring out the best in your child. And your ability to redesign a ritual that is attuned to the changing demands of growing children is itself among the hallmarks of a healthy family.

There is one feeding challenge that cuts across all ages and stages, from nursing a baby to feeding an elderly parent: when your carefully prepared meal is rejected. Food and love are so intertwined that it takes a strong parental ego not to feel that you are being rejected when a child refuses your food. But there are so many reasons for a child to turn away from a food offering, reasons that have nothing to do with loving you.

The child might not be hungry because she doesn't feel well or because she's been snacking all afternoon. She might not like the smell of the food, or she may want to express her autonomy by taking control of her eating, or she may want to make life harder for you because she's angry with you or with another child who looked at her cross-eyed on the playground. My point is that food refusal is not a battle to get into with your child. Better to find a peaceful moment later in the day to ask calmly about it, and see if you can come up with ideas to make dinner more appetizing. Or just let it go, and try again tomorrow.

THE FIRST DINNERS: IN THE WOMB AND AT THE BREAST

None of us can remember our very first family dinners. I'm thinking about the meals we had in the dark, cozy confines of the womb, swallowing amniotic fluids, which actually transmit the flavors of chicken curry or matzo ball soup, or whatever our mother had eaten for dinner. There is mounting evidence to support the claim that a mother's diet during pregnancy paves the way for her baby's first food preferences.[1] Those in utero slurps of flavored amniotic fluid make babies predisposed to liking the same flavors once they are out of the womb. For example, babies who had repeated exposure to carrot juice during the last trimester of pregnancy had positive facial expressions when they first tried carrot-flavored cereal—"Oh yeah, I remember this yummy taste."

The wider the range of foods the pregnant mother eats, the more foods the baby will recognize.[2] My craving for chopped-chicken-liver sandwiches during my first pregnancy may account for my first son's passion for corned beef with chicken livers; likewise, my avoidance of fish because it made me feel queasy during my second pregnancy might explain my younger son's early distaste for most fish dishes. Indeed, the foods that one eats during pregnancy can influence one's child's receptivity to those foods.

The mother's role as shaper of her baby's palate continues during breastfeeding. A mother's milk actually takes on the flavors of the food she eats. She creates a bridge from what she eats to what her baby tastes. Since children prefer foods that are familiar, the flavors that babies taste over and over again in their mother's milk will be their earliest experience of familiar flavors and will likely influence the foods that they gravitate toward when they are offered those same foods in solid form. It is no wonder that preferences for certain cultural foods get laid down during pregnancy and breastfeeding.

Fathers also play a critical role in early feeding. They can provide regular bottles of breast-pumped milk, or of formula, offering a welcome break to a nursing mother. Most important, when fathers leave all the feeding to women, they miss out on one of the coziest, most satisfying parts of taking care of a baby. And feeling left out of the mother-baby dyad feeds its own resentment, so it's better to figure out a way for both parents to participate in the warm bonding that takes place during feeding.

Regardless of whether a baby is bottle or breast-fed (by mother or father, or both) the feeding relationship is the first crucial task of parenting. When feeding is warm and consistent, it creates a building block for later feelings of attachment. Babies learn they can count on you to take care of their needs. And, since feeding is a reciprocal process, it's the first place that your baby learns about his impact on you. When he cries, he can get you to feed him. Through a predictable, reliable feeding experience, your baby learns that the world is a safe place. Other caregivers—babysitters, grandparents, daycare staff—also play an important role in creating a warm feeding experience, and they help widen your baby's understanding of the world as a trustworthy place.

There are many behaviors that help support a positive feeding experience: looking at your baby, holding your baby securely, letting her decide when to eat, how much to have and when to stop, and all this without a lot of interruptions to wipe or burp her. Once your child is about six months old, it is important to let her decide how much to eat and to self-feed. It's a positive experience for your child to get messy—although I know the cleanup is no fun when she's making her food into a train track with locomotives going across her high chair—so talk to her in a quiet but encouraging manner. But this is only the first opportunity to make eating enjoyable.

There will be lots of other points along the way to direct the train toward a satisfying dinner.

HOW TO MAKE YOUR TODDLER AN ADVENTUROUS EATER

Young kids are not the most civilized dinner companions. Dinnertime can feel like sitting with a group of monkeys who like to throw and smear their food, and have short attention spans once they finish eating. This is a critical time, however, for both parents and children to develop family meals as a ritual. One researcher of family rituals found that by the time kids are preschool age, if parents find little meaning in their daily rituals, they are also less satisfied with their marriages.[3] Plus, when children are toddlers, they are more receptive to trying new foods than are children age four to eight. So the preschool years provide a time of great opportunity to get a dinner ritual started and to offer your child many new foods.

While children are toddlers, parents play a key role in encouraging adventurous eating. An effective strategy to prevent picky eating is for parents to model their own enjoyment of foods they are offering their kids at the dinner table. Less effective is for parents to restrict foods or to pressure their kids to eat. If you want your children to try new foods, don't tell them they're not allowed to have dessert unless they eat all their vegetables. In a recent study, researchers found that when parents used rewards to encourage food tasting or dismissed a child's expression of hunger or fullness, the children were almost twice as likely not to eat fruits and vegetables.[4] A better way is to eat the new food with gusto in front of your children, and then ask, "Would you like to taste it?" You could ask your child to tell you a few words to describe the taste. This focuses your child's attention on the food, rather than on rejecting it. Also, serving food "family style" in bowls or platters placed on the table allows children to see the adults enjoying a food that the kids can just reach out and try.

ENROLL YOUR YOUNG KIDS AS SOUS-CHEFS

Toddlers will want to be right in the kitchen with you while you are making dinner. Having a low cabinet with a few old pots and pans, wooden spoons, and empty squeeze bottles can keep kids occupied for hours. Or putting a chair up at the sink to allow them to play with soap, eyedroppers, sponges, and plastic buckets can also keep them busy. A young child can also "make" a parallel meal by taking discarded vegetable scraps and mixing them together alongside you.

For young children, actually sitting down and eating dinner might be less important than the fun of helping to create it. Preschoolers, after all, are as interested in the journey as the destination, are as invested in helping to make the meal as in eating it. When you take a walk with them, they may want to pause to look at a piece of trash or stop to pet a dog. They usually don't march straight ahead intent on arriving at their destination as quickly as possible. So it is with mealtime. The whole process of mixing, stirring, and making a mess fascinates young children. The whirring machines in the kitchen may also be captivating. My son Joe was obsessed with kitchen machines as a toddler, running to the KitchenAid mixer as soon as he woke up in the morning to tell me with a gesture, since he didn't have the words, that he wanted to beat some eggs. We ate meringues, soufflés, and brownies at least once a day for a year. I would have had an easier time setting limits on this behavior if I also didn't have a huge sweet tooth.

Of course, there will be many evenings when you just want to get the food on the table as quickly as possible, and having a mess-generating sous-chef will be annoying. There might be other nights when it is relaxing to cook dinner in a quiet kitchen while your partner entertains or bathes the children somewhere else. But one of the great joys of having toddlers in the kitchen is their willingness to jump in and help—and some recipes particularly lend themselves to young children.

Susan Swick is a child psychiatrist and the mother of four children under the age of eight. At her house, the dinner meal starts while she is cooking and can last for an hour and a half, even if the sit-down part of the meal is only ten or fifteen minutes. By encouraging her children to cook alongside her, she extends the time she spends with them, and she gets them involved and interested in the meal. As an extra bonus, a child's participation in making the meal usually guarantees that the child is invested in wanting to eat his own creation. A young cook might even try to entice his siblings into trying the dish.

One favorite all-hands-on family dinner at the Swick-Troekel house is Origami Dumplings (see page 30). If I hadn't witnessed this family making these dumplings, I wouldn't have believed that such a multistep recipe with so many kids was possible. I don't think I could have pulled this off with my two children when they were so young. But the kids had a lot of fun, and the results were delicious.

Eight-year-old Jacob and five-year-old Lily stuffed the square wrappers with carrots, cabbage, and tofu, and then folded each one in a different origami-like creation to resemble a boat, a hat, or an animal. Meanwhile, four-year-old Minha nibbled at the stuffing while stirring together carrot shavings and broccoli scraps with a little water to make her own concoction. One-year-old Luke ate the cooked vegetables in the dumpling stuffing, and his older brother and sisters fed him in his high chair. The dumplings are a complete meal of vegetables and protein—a crowd-pleaser for all ages.

The main challenge at this stage of development is making a dinner that will appeal to both your young children and to grown-ups, since the last thing you want to do is make multiple meals. It's also important to manage your expectations so that you don't get discouraged if dinner is over in a flash. You are setting down the foundation by establishing a ritual that your child will grow into. A few basic principles can help:

- Create meals that have some flexibility built into them. For example, you can roll some chicken tenders in breadcrumbs and Parmesan cheese for the kids. Then, as Laurie Colwin wrote in her book *Home Cooking,* you can also mix up some mustard with crushed garlic, a dash of cinnamon, and a pinch of cayenne pepper. Slather this mixture on some other chicken tenders and roll in breadcrumbs. Dab all of the chicken with a little butter, and pop it into a 375-degree oven. At the end of one hour, the kids will have tasty cheesy chicken, and the parents will have a somewhat spicier version.

- Don't underestimate your toddler's taste buds. The idea that young children and adults must eat different foods might be a myth created by marketers and food manufacturers. After all, the food industry stands to make more money if parents believe that their children

A RECIPE TO MAKE WITH PRESCHOOLERS

ORIGAMI DUMPLINGS

(Courtesy of Dr. Susan Swick and Dr. Matt Troekel)

1 (8-ounce) package firm tofu, drained (wrap it in a dish towel
     on a plate with a pot or other weight on top for about
     20 minutes)
1 tablespoon Asian five-spice powder
2 to 3 tablespoons peanut or canola oil, divided
1 to 2 garlic cloves, minced
1 tablespoon minced fresh ginger
1 to 1½ cups each of finely chopped vegetables, such as green
     cabbage, carrots, mushrooms, zucchini, and broccoli
1 (12-ounce) package dumpling wrappers (for smaller fingers,
     use egg roll wrappers, which are larger)
Oil for frying
Store-bought dumpling dipping sauce or soy sauce

Cut the drained tofu into small cubes (the size of dice) and toss in a
bowl with the Asian five-spice.

Add enough oil to a wok or frying pan to fully coat the bottom
with a thick layer. Heat the oil. Fry the tofu, stirring often so it doesn't
stick. It may crumble but that doesn't matter. Remove the tofu from
the pan when it is lightly browned.

In the same pan, heat additional oil. Fry the garlic and ginger until
the garlic is browned but not burnt. Then add the vegetables, starting
with the crunchiest (which takes longer to cook). As one vegetable
starts to look tender, add the next one. Toss and sample often to know
when it is tender enough to eat easily.

Turn off the heat and add the tofu, mixing everything together in
the pan. Transfer the mixture to a bowl.

It's dumpling building time! Give everyone a stack of dumpling
wrappers and a spoon. Also put out a plate, a dish of water, and a bowl

of filling. Spoon a small amount of filling into the center of a wrapper. Use your finger to place water where you will attach one side of the dumpling to the other, like glue on an envelope flap. Try any shape you can imagine. (Parents tend to make a lot of simple triangles, which are most stable and hold the most filling, while the kids make purses, hats, jungle animals, etc.)

To **fry** the dumplings, cook in 1 to 2 inches of oil in a large frying pan at a very high heat. This is messy, but it's the preferred taste for many (crispy, if done right).

To **boil** the dumplings, bring a large pot of water to a boil and then drop the dumplings into the water. Simmer for about 12 minutes (Boiling tends to make the dumplings soft and doughy and can result in many exploded dumplings.)

To **steam** the dumplings, spray cooking oil on a vegetable steamer (this is very important; otherwise, they stick and rip). Place the steamer in a large pot. (The pot needs to have a lid, and it must be deep enough to be taller than the steamer and the dumplings.) Add just enough water to the pot under the steamer so it doesn't come in contact with the dumplings. Place the dumplings on the steamer; add the lid. Boil the water. Pour a little water over the dumplings once or twice during the next 5 minutes. The dumpling skins should contract and look shiny when they're finished. Steaming gives a firm and chewy dumpling.

Enjoy the dumplings with dipping sauce or soy sauce (and chopsticks, if you're brave). The fun is to see if you can figure out whose dumpling you are eating!

need brightly colored cereals and lunches packaged with toys than if parents and children can enjoy the same real food together.
- One pediatrician I interviewed about family dinners advised that young children should never be given "separator plates" because it makes them grow up thinking that foods shouldn't touch. Then, they may shun dishes like stews and salads and want only plain pasta.

- Involve toddlers in the meal preparation. Pulling basil leaves off stems, spinning salad greens, plopping chopped vegetables into a salad or a pan, smelling a spice, setting the timer, tasting the soup to see if it needs more salt, sprinkling cheese on vegetables, mashing cooked vegetables, and turning on and off a food processor are some of the many things that young children can do.
- Ask young children to flip through a cookbook and choose a dinner they would like to help with. Mollie Katzen's *Honest Pretzels* and *Pretend Soup,* and Sally Sampson's *ChopChop* offer recipes that are appealing and accessible to young kids.
- Play is the work of childhood, so you may want to provide toddlers with ways to play with food. One example is to ask your child to ar-

---

HOW TO KEEP YOUNG KIDS AT THE TABLE

- Give them ice pops made with fresh juice. It will take young kids about five minutes to finish one pop. This is a useful tip for breakfast as well as dinner. My husband did this at every breakfast so that he could read the newspaper for a few extra minutes.
- Ask your child to guess the ingredients in each dish, and include a secret ingredient (like a dash of cinnamon or a splash of soy sauce).
- Invite your child to stir a pot, crumble the cheese, or set the timer—having a hand in making the meal creates pride and ownership.
- Avoid having a revolving door at the dinner table. If your child wants to leave the table, let him, but perhaps only once. After two departures he should know that his dinnertime is over.
- Present each part of the meal as a course. For example, peas as an appetizer, pasta with pesto sauce as the main course, and orange slices for dessert.
- Play a word game at the table: "I ran into someone in the supermarket today. Can you ask yes-or-no questions to guess who it was?" or "Close your eyes. Can you remember the color of the walls, what color shirt your father is wearing, or where you left your backpack?" (See Chapter 6 for more games to play at the table with toddlers.)

range cut-up vegetables as a face on each family member's plate. (See Chapter 5 for more ideas.)

- Avoid letting food became an area of struggle over who has power. Food is an area where kids assert power when they don't have power in other parts of their lives, and most young children don't wield all that much power (other than the occasional public temper tantrum when parents may be willing to concede to any demands to get this to stop). Letting your children have choices at the table and in other areas of their lives will make food less charged. For example, if your child refuses to eat a particular meal, it's best to stay calm and not send her away from the table. You might offer her an alternative, such as cereal with milk, a bowl of yogurt, or a peanut butter and jelly sandwich—choices, yes, but nothing too exciting, and nothing that makes too much extra work for you.

- If your child insists on eating the same foods, like pasta, night after night, roll with it. You can offer many vegetables, fruits, and protein as "sides" or even mixed in with the pasta. Just keep offering new foods, and try not to get discouraged. For everyone's sanity, you don't want to make mealtime a big struggle, and in the context of a relaxed dinner, a child will be much more likely to try new foods.

DINNER WITH SCHOOL-AGE KIDS: ADDING COMPETENCE AND RULES INTO THE MIX

The years between six and twelve are about learning to share and compromise—lessons that your children will absorb in the classroom, on the playground, and around the dinner table. Just as kids are learning that they cannot always get their own way when choosing a game to play at recess, they will learn at home that not everyone gets their choice of meal every night. You may find that your kids want the meal choice to be "fair," each child getting to choose one meal a week, for example, or each getting the chance to veto one proposed meal. Children will want "airtime" at the dinner table to be equitably distributed as well, although more reserved children might need coaxing to tell a story about their day.

As children become more aware of the world around them, they might start to ask for foods they have seen advertised on TV or clamor for foods they have eaten at their friends' houses. At this time your family's identity as distinct and different from others can emerge, and what you serve at dinner can be one of the defining features. Some of my sons' friends liked to come over for spicy sesame noodles or apple-and-cheese crepes, while my sons coveted the brisket at one friend's house and the traditional Chinese *jook* at a neighbor's.

When children are school-age, it becomes harder to protect them from the onslaught of marketing aimed at enticing them to consume fatty foods, soft drinks, and other unhealthy treats. It's also the easiest time to engage them in eating dinner with their parents. (Indeed, more than half of nine-year-olds eat dinner with their families every day, compared to only a third of fourteen-year-olds.)[5]

As they progress through elementary school, girls and boys become competent to read and follow recipes. They can help with setting the table, clearing their places, and aiding in the cleanup. Their involvement in the dinner ritual contributes to their interest in it. At this stage, my kids wanted to be more involved in cooking, an impulse I encouraged. One of their favorite games was to create a restaurant with tablecloths, menus that they printed, and a pad to take orders. They would send me out to do their shopping and then would let me hang around as a sous-chef while they created their own concoctions.

MAKING DINNERS THAT ENGAGE SIX- TO TWELVE-YEAR-OLD KIDS

One challenge at this stage is your child's increasing awareness of the outside world, and with it the idea that there are other foods to eat besides the ones in their house. It's also a time to harness the school-age child's wish to be more competent and to play by the rules. Here are few developmentally informed guidelines to keep in mind:

- Since school-age kids like structure and order, they may feel comforted by a predictable schedule of meals. For example, in my sister's family, Tuesday night was seafood, Wednesday was chicken, Thursday was tacos, Friday night pasta with pesto and chicken sausages, and so on. This routine cuts down on conflict if your children can agree on five or six meals. Often, this routine needs to be tweaked or altered to prevent boredom or to accommodate new tastes or the demands of a new season.

- At this stage of development, kids are very interested in foods they have seen advertised on TV or eaten in restaurants. It can be fun to re-create one of these meals at home. For example, most supermarkets offer ready-made pizza dough. It's simple to roll it out on a floured surface, and then place it on an oiled cookie sheet. Spread on tomato sauce from a jar, and customize the pizza with mushrooms, peppers, onions, sliced pepperoni, eggplant, or anything else that appeals to you and your kids. Sprinkle Parmesan or mozzarella cheese (or both) on top, and bake for about 10 minutes in a 450-degree oven. Other restaurant-type meals that translate easily into home kitchens are tacos (see the recipe on page 100) and crepes (see the recipe on page 36).

- This is a time when kids are getting more involved in activities outside the house, so finding a regular time and place for dinner can present a challenge. Family dinners sometimes happen on a ball field, in the stands of a basketball court, or backstage at a play rehearsal. It's better to be flexible about bringing a picnic that everyone can partake of than to give up on dinner altogether. One building block for a portable meal is Asian chicken wings (see the recipe on p. 37).

- Do a role reversal one night a week when you have your children do the cooking. In our house, I went to a meeting every other Thursday night. On those nights, from the time my sons were ten and twelve, they did the cooking, always making some kind of beef, lamb, or pork dish—foods I never made.

- Invite your children to practice resistance to destructive media messages. Ask children why they think TV ads are advertising processed food in a plastic container rather than carrots and celery. Or ask them what would happen if junk food carried a high tax the way cigarettes do. Or what it would be like if their school refused to sell unhealthy food in the cafeteria.

RECIPE FOR SCHOOL-AGE KIDS AND THEIR PARENTS

CREPES (FOR 4)

(Adapted from *Joy of Cooking*)

These can be made in about 35 minutes. The batter is very quick to prepare, and while it's congealing in the refrigerator for 30 minutes you and your kids can be making the filling. (I invested in a crepe pan, since it gave the whole venture more authenticity and made it a more special dinner. But, really, any nonstick pan will work just fine.)

Batter:
   ½ cup all-purpose flour
   ½ cup milk
   ¼ cup lukewarm water
   2 large eggs
   2 tablespoons melted butter
   Pinch of salt

Combine all the ingredients in a blender or food processor. Put the batter into a covered container and place in the refrigerator for at least 30 minutes.

Filling Suggestions:
   Sautéed vegetables and grated Swiss cheese
   Sautéed apples and grated cheddar cheese

Directions:
Melt a small dollop of butter in a crepe pan or small frying pan.
   Remove the batter from the refrigerator and stir it well. Pour about ¼ cup batter onto the hot pan, swirling the pan to coat evenly. Cook until little bubbles form and the underside is golden. Then flip the crepe, using your fingers or a spatula. Cook until the second side is light brown.

Remove the crepe from the pan and place on wax paper. Repeat until you have at least one crepe per person.

Invite family members to assemble their own by placing the desired filling down the middle of the crepe. Then fold each side of the crepe to the middle.

ASIAN CHICKEN WINGS (FOR 6 TO 8)

1 cup soy sauce

½ cup olive oil

5 garlic cloves, minced

1 chunk ginger, minced

2 tablespoons dark brown sugar

4 to 5 pounds chicken wings

Whisk together the soy sauce, olive oil, garlic, ginger, and brown sugar. Pour over the chicken wings, and let marinate for at least 30 minutes (or overnight).

Preheat the oven to 400 degrees. Place the wings on a cookie sheet lined with aluminum foil (for easier cleanup), and bake for 45 minutes. Remove the wings from the oven, flip them over, and bake for about 40 minutes longer.

These wings are delicious at any temperature and tend to draw kids from other families to join you. They are like catnip at a sporting event.

You can bring a pasta salad or cut-up veggies and fruits and you have a well-balanced meal. Just pack a lot of napkins because the wings are messy.

DINNER WITH ADOLESCENTS

Adolescence is a time of exploration in the context of ongoing connection with the family. Kids are discovering new music and new friends, experimenting with their sexual identities and their appearances, but still using home as their touchstone.

Family researchers have identified several features of successful parents of adolescents. They are interested in their kids' journeys and want to learn about their kids' new discoveries; they are tolerant of strong expressions of feelings; and they are willing to talk in a more honest and self-disclosing way about their own lives, if these disclosures are relevant to their kids' struggles.[6] This is also a time when kids are figuring out who they are and how they want to be similar to and different from their parents. It's no wonder then that this is a time when kids may declare that they have food preferences that are unlike those of their parents. Consider the *New Yorker* cartoon of two teenage girls talking. One says to the other: "I started to be a vegetarian for health reasons, now it's just to annoy!" Or conversely, my son Joe started cooking meat when he was about thirteen, an act that simultaneously delighted his father and differentiated him from me.

How to Keep Dinner as Lively as Your Teenagers

Some of the following suggestions may fall flat as a pancake. Others might only get you a few more minutes of conversation at the table. Still others might not work the first or second time you try them. When it comes to parenting teens, persistence pays off—so does having a thick skin when your teen rolls his eyes at you. Don't let a little pushback or negativity keep you from trying again.

- Agree that dinner is off-limits for discussing conflicts—no talk about homework, whose turn it is to take out the trash, a recent D on a math quiz, or how late curfew should be on Friday night.
- Eliminating dicey content, however, will not eliminate all conflict at the table. Most teenagers can find things to wrangle about no matter how friendly the topics of conversation seem to you. My kids often got into tussles with one another over who was taking up more physical space at the table. Teenagers can get fights going over the size of a plate or the tone of your voice. Try asking everyone to hit the pause button: "Let's all take a deep breath or step away from the table for a minute." Alternatively, you can ask your child if there is anything

that's irritating him or making him feel prickly at the moment, other than the color of the drinking glasses. Assure him that you really are interested.

- If possible, parents as well as teens should make dinner a technology-free zone. If this isn't possible, then negotiate rules that everyone can agree to, such as: "We'll only use our phones to resolve factual disagreements that come up at dinner."

- If scheduling conflicts are interfering with dinners—what with sport practices, after-school jobs, hours of homework, and heavy social media upkeep—consider having a healthy after-dinner, take-a-break-from homework snack. This might be frozen yogurt with berries, a bowl of soup, or cheese and crackers.

- Initiate conversations about subjects that matter to all of you, such as an article in the newspaper that confused, upset, or delighted you. Talk about it and ask for your kids' reactions.

- Tell a story about something that you struggled with during the day and invite your children to help solve a dilemma you faced, such as needing to give mixed feedback to someone at work, or sending an unintended email and having to repair the repercussions.

- Offer to make a new meal, based on your teen's interests—if he is studying South African history or Indian literature, check out Epicurious.com online and search for recipes by country. Even better, make that new meal with your child so that she can teach you something about another culture she knows more about than you do.

- Invite your kid to make a course or part of the meal, particularly something fairly quick (but special and dramatic) that will elicit oohs and ahs from the rest of the family—popovers, bananas flambé, and fruit smoothies all do the trick.

- Speak about your own experiences of the day in a way that is honest and self-disclosing, perhaps revealing something that was embarrassing or challenging. Or repeat a joke that you heard at work.

- Create a weekly dinner ritual when your kids' friends or family are invited to dinner or to dessert. For example, on a tired Sunday night, invite friends over to make sundaes.

- Ask your teen to choose music for you to listen to during dinner. On other nights, you might play your own music, or play the music that you listened to when you were your child's age. This will also provide something interesting to discuss.
- Since adolescence is a time of increased exploration, buy cookbooks when you travel to new places, or ask for recipes at restaurants, or from people you meet. We love to make a meal that conjures up a trip to Italy—a pasta recipe from a friend we made in Rome who invited us to have this meal at her home (see box "A Recipe That Captures a Family Adventure").

EMPTY-NEST DINNERS

Family dinners don't stop when adolescents leave home. Some couples with an empty nest observe that dinnertime continues to be a placeholder, a time when they still feel connected to their kids as they eat a favorite family meal or say a blessing that they have said for decades. Some couples also report a newfound flexibility: "We can have dinner at nine o'clock if we like," or "It's so much easier to cook a meal without having to take into account my children's food preferences."

It took me years after my children flew the coop not to feel wistful around dinnertime, though at first my husband and I pretended that this new freedom was great. We sometimes had leftovers two nights in a row, something that would have elicited grumbles from our sons. Other times, we misbehaved like children, snacking on cheese and crackers until we lost our appetites for dinner. Eventually, we settled into a new rhythm of eating at more varied times of the night than we used to, and eating way down the food chain. My omnivore husband has inexplicably become a vegetarian three or four nights a week.

For some empty nesters, dinner can feel like an awkward time, as it is a poignant and nightly reminder that family life is forever changed. One couple found that they turned on the nightly news at dinnertime, a practice that was verboten when their children were home. They realized that with the TV on they were trying to find a substitute for the liveliness of their

A RECIPE THAT CAPTURES A FAMILY ADVENTURE

MARINA'S PASTA WITH SHRIMP AND CLAMS (FOR 4 TO 6)

1 garlic clove, minced

1 onion, chopped

2 tablespoons olive oil

8 ounces white wine

20 cherry tomatoes

¾ pound shrimp

About 20 small clams in their shells

1 pound linguini

2 tablespoons chopped parsley

Boil water in a large pot to prepare to cook the pasta. While the water is boiling, brown the garlic and onion in olive oil in a large saucepan.

Add the wine and the tomatoes to the pan, and simmer for about 10 minutes.

Add the shrimp and cook for about 2 minutes. Set the pan aside.

Boil about an inch of water in a large frying pan. Reduce the heat to simmer and add the clams. Stir the clams in the water, removing each one as it opens. Discard any clams that did not open. Filter the broth with a cloth placed over a colander. Save the broth.

Remove the clams from their shells and add them plus 1 cup of the broth to the pan with the shrimp. Keep warm.

Cook the pasta in the pot of boiling water and drain when it is *al dente,* reserving a small amount of pasta water. Add the pasta and the small amount of pasta water to the pan with the sauce. Sprinkle with parsley just before serving.

children's conversation. With that insight, they decided to keep it on just when they were preparing dinner but would try to allow their own adult conversation to develop at the table.

WHEN YOUNG ADULT CHILDREN COME HOME

And, of course college kids and older ones continue to come home during vacations and school breaks. They may want you to prepare a sentimental favorite or they may be interested in what new dishes you've experimented with in their absence. Food is so synonymous with home that an adult child can experience a longing for home as a longing for a home-cooked meal. A friend of mine told me that she came home from work one day and could sense that someone had been in her kitchen, even though it was totally clean. She was right. Her nineteen-year-old son, a college sophomore, had let himself in because he yearned for a home-cooked meal. Turns out, he wanted the taste of a home-cooked meal, cooked by him.

Dinner with young adult children can also give a taste of a new shift in roles. When my son, Gabe, came home for the summer at age twenty-two, after graduating from college and taking a trip to Vietnam, I thought we would slide into the comfortable dinner-making patterns of his childhood. Instead, he took the lead in the kitchen that summer, and this has been the pattern ever since.

It began when he offered to teach me how to make the spring roll recipe that he had learned at the Hai Café cooking school in Hoi An, Vietnam. I offered to shop for the ingredients. With time short, I had to make several substitutions. Instead of taro root (which my son used gloves to handle in Vietnam so as not to develop an itchy rash), I got a turnip. Instead of choko, which I couldn't find at the supermarket, I bought chayote from Costa Rica, a similar yellow squash. Instead of wood ear mushrooms, I got dried black trumpet mushrooms. Still, even with all these short cuts and westernizations, the spring rolls were the most delicious I had ever tasted. (See the recipe on page 43.)

Those spring rolls were just the start. Instead of the slapped-together roast chicken that I made throughout his childhood, the epitome of comfort food, Gabe has figured out how to butterfly a chicken. I still don't know how to do this, but I can attest to the results: The chicken is far juicier than my old-fashioned roast chicken.

During my sons' growing up years, I was usually the one trying new things in the kitchen. Now the roles are reversed. Perhaps, part of the compensation for having children leave home is that sometimes they return, willing to share their adventures with us.

SPRING ROLLS, HOI AN STYLE (FOR 4)

(Adapted from the Hai Café Cooking School, Hoi An, Vietnam)

1 cup finely chopped vermicelli noodles, softened in cold water

⅓ pound shrimp, sliced down the middle and then cut in half

1 cup finely chopped black trumpet mushrooms, softened in warm water

1 cup julienned green beans

1 cup thinly diced shallots

1 cup finely grated carrots

1 cup finely grated chayote

1 cup finely grated turnip

1 large egg yolk

1 pinch salt

1 pinch pepper

½ cup vegetable oil (not more than 1 inch deep in frying pan)

1 packet 8.5-ounce round rice paper sheets, softened in water. (You need 1½ sheets for each roll.)

In a large mixing bowl, combine the noodles, shrimp, mushrooms, beans, shallots, carrots, chayote, turnip, egg yolk, salt, and pepper; mix well.

Place 1 sheet of rice paper on the counter, and then put half of another sheet on the part closest to you. Place about 2 tablespoons of the mixture on the paper that has double thickness. Then roll it up, taking care to tuck in the sides as you roll. Repeat to use the entire filling, which will make about 12 spring rolls. Prick each roll with a fork to help them cook well.

Heat the oil in a large frying pan. Place the spring rolls into the oil; turn once when they are golden on one side. Remove from the pan, and drain on paper towels. Serve with Fish Sauce.

Fish Sauce:

    2 tablespoons bottled fish sauce

    1 teaspoon crushed garlic

    1 teaspoon finely chopped jalapeño chili pepper

    1 teaspoon sugar

    1 tablespoon lime or lemon juice

Combine all the ingredients in a small bowl and mix thoroughly until the sugar dissolves.

DINNER WITH OLDER FAMILY MEMBERS

For a variety of reasons, it's increasingly difficult for elderly people to eat well. But eating well is just as important at this stage of life as it is for the young. In fact, eating well may be the single best predictor of being able to live independently.

There are many physical changes associated with aging that alter our relationship to food. Between the ages of sixty and eighty our sense of taste and smell decrease. Because older people also have decreased sensitivity to the sensations of hunger and thirst, they sometimes forget to eat or stay hydrated. The threshold for taste rises with age, so older eaters often need more flavor and seasonings to enjoy their meals. Appetite also takes a hit when a frail or mostly sedentary person lacks the energy to participate in physical activity. And the reverse is true too: With less food, people have less energy for activity. One change that might expand the options for older eaters is that sensitivity to disgust wanes with age. Maybe by the time I turn eighty, my sons can take me out on the town for a dinner that features raw eggs with uncooked pork sausage, a dinner that now makes me want to gag.

Elderly people's living situations can contribute to diminished eating. In general, married couples eat better than singles. Perhaps, when you have someone to share your meals with, it's easier to remember to cook—and to want to eat. Living alone—like two-thirds of women and one-third of men over the age of seventy-five—correlates with skipped meals. Assisted living facilities that provide healthy food and opportunities to eat with others can create a new kind of family dinner. Many elderly people I've worked with tell me that the best part of moving into a retirement community is that they don't have to cook anymore and they never have to eat alone.

Given that with age comes a dimming of taste and smell, it's the pleasing appearance of the meal and the way it evokes memories of food and family that will stimulate appetite. When you're cooking for elderly relatives or friends, it's good to pay special attention to the color of foods and to the evocative power of a dish to stimulate a sluggish appetite.

When my elderly father joined us for dinner, I tried to make foods that reminded him of happy memories. For example, I might make a baked apple, a favorite food from his childhood, or sweet potato pudding, a dish that evoked his wife (and my mother) who used to make this dish for every holiday. Even with the diminishing of taste buds in old age, food continues to be a source of great enjoyment. M. F. K. Fisher, a food writer, mused about the appetite during old age: "For many people, eating is the only pleasure left, as were the endless dishes and unceasing cups of wine to the aged Ulysses. . . . But, we must grow old, and we must eat."[7]

At any age, it is the infusion of meaning that adds extra flavor to a meal. At infancy, the flavor comes from the warm feelings of closeness and attachment; for toddlers, the flavor is imbued through the fun of playing with food; for school-age kids, the boost to flavor comes from feeling more competent to participate in meal preparation; during adolescence, dinner is tastier when it is as much about being with the family as asserting a separate identity; with young adults the meaning often comes from being able to go home again, and sometimes in being able to teach your parents a thing or two.

PART TWO

......

THE MAIN
COURSE

Food, Fun, and

Conversation

4

Tips for Healthy Eating

I f you're eating a nightly family meal at home, you already have a leg up on healthy eating. When we eat at home rather than in a restaurant, food portions tend to be more reasonably sized, and fruits and vegetables are more reliably offered. Sodas and high-fat foods, like French fries, are also less likely to show up at home than if the meal is eaten at a restaurant. It's not just that eating family dinner gives kids a health boost, but what they learn about food at dinner translates to their other meals.

Many people find it difficult to figure out how to make a healthy meal, but it's not as hard as you might think it is. Parents are often confused and overwhelmed by all the food choices at the supermarket—about 45,000 items on offer, with about 20,000 new products introduced each year.[1] And there is too much food grown each year in America—almost 3,900 calories per day for every man, woman, and child, even though the average adult needs only about 2,200 calories and children require even fewer. Food companies deal with this overabundance by advertising snack foods, offering larger portions, and getting families to eat more by making food more convenient and cheaper. Another way they increase food consumption is by offering more options. In a study where adults were offered unlimited access to M&M's, people ate more of these candies when there were a greater variety of colors presented.[2]

It's not just that we are being marketed lots of unhealthy foods but we are also exposed to a shifting, confusing landscape of diets and food fads. Should I get low fat or low carbs for my family? Is butter a better fat than margarine, or is it vice-versa? How often do I need to feed my family broccoli to get the anti-cancer properties I've read about? Is coffee going to increase my risk of pancreatic cancer or decrease my risk of Alzheimer's?

As Ellen Goodman, a former *Boston Globe* columnist, wryly noted, "There seems to be some sort of planned obsolescence now to medical news. Today's cure is tomorrow's poison pellet. Fresh research has a sell-by date that is shorter than the one on the cereal box."[3]

Indeed, information about nutrition should be taken with a grain of salt, sugar, and fat. For starters, nutritional science is a relatively young field that doesn't yet explain what happens inside our bodies when we eat different foods. But the newness of proven scientific findings doesn't prevent "news" about nutrition from being reported quite vigorously and quickly, in ways that, let's say, news about astrophysics or molecular biology isn't. Nutrition news, when it's based only on a single study involving mice, or with the participation of only a very small group of people, makes for catchy headlines. Take these, plucked recently from Science Daily, an online website:

- "High salt consumption appears to be bad for your bones."
- "Adolescents' high fat diet impairs memory and learning."
- "A few cups of hot cocoa may help fight obesity-related inflammation."
- "Vegetarian diets associated with lower risk of death."[4]

Some of these findings may well stand up when the studies are repeated over time. Some, however, have been done on animals only and don't necessarily apply to humans.

But even studies done on humans are fallible, since diets change from week to week, and certainly year to year. How many of us are eating the same dinners now as we did a few years ago, despite children having grown up, a favorite grocery store closing, a discovery of a new ethnic cuisine, and eating out more or less as finances change?

Nutrition studies also may depend on *reports* of what respondents ate in a given week. (Do you remember what you ate for lunch yesterday?) And, finally, it's very difficult to apply the gold standard of research to nutrition studies. That would require researchers to randomly assign one group of individuals to eat a set diet, measured out for them, over several years, while another group ate another diet, similarly measured but with the items in question, such as calcium, high fats, or meat, removed.

Nevertheless, while there may be no scientific consensus about the merits of eating a particular food to prevent a particular illness, there are some broad strokes that are well documented by researchers. In general, the health status of American children has actually improved over the last thirty years in terms of lowered rates of infant mortality and declines in nutrient deficiencies of the past, like rickets. But, the rates of overweight kids dramatically increased from the 1980s until 2000.[5]

However, recently, childhood obesity rates have plateaued, or even declined slightly in developed countries, particularly among preschool children (ages two to five).[6] This positive trend is probably attributable to public health programs and growing public awareness of the need for physical activity and the harm of TV watching and soft drink consumption.[7] Despite this glimmer of good news, two-thirds of children age two to eight are not consuming the recommended number of servings of fruits, and three-quarters of those youngsters are falling behind in their consumption of recommended vegetables. And about three-quarters of American children exceed the dietary recommendations for total or saturated fats.[8] According to the American Dietetic Association's 2014 review, too many American children are eating diets that do not meet the minimum recommendations for a healthy diet.[9]

The reasons for this substandard state of affairs are also well documented. American kids are eating more of their food at fast-food restaurants and as snack foods, both pathways to higher fat and sugar consumption. About 40 percent of family food dollars are now spent on food eaten outside of the home.[10]

Michael Pollan, a writer and journalism professor, blames our Western diet, as it has manifested over the last few decades, for the rise in obesity, cancer, heart disease, and diabetes in Americans. Specifically, he targets the focus on highly processed foods and refined grains, the use of chemicals to raise plants and animals for food, an overabundance of sugar and fat, and a narrowing of biological diversity in favor of growing a few plentiful, hardy crops—particularly soy, corn and wheat.[11]

Mindful that there is much we don't know, I offer some suggestions to help parents make sense of the confusing landscape of food choices. Drawing on interviews with pediatricians and nutritionists, as well as on the research from Marion Nestle and Michael Pollan, I have culled the best advice available to make dinner as healthy as possible without becoming a battlefield for calorie-counters and fat-fighters. Parents need help, both in simplifying the known data and understanding what isn't yet known, so that they don't get bogged down in the latest food fad.

SERVE A VARIETY OF HEALTHY FOODS

Different vegetables and fruits confer unique benefits to our immune systems and to the health of different organs, such as our skin, eyes, and liver. As one pediatrician told me: "A colorful plate is a healthy plate. Colors are better for you, while white foods tend to be less good." Pollan offers the same advice: "Eat your colors."

INVITE YOUR CHILDREN TO TRY NEW FOODS

It's much more fun to cook for a family that is willing to try new things, but getting children to eat new foods is often easier said than done. Children, particularly those from ages three to eight, can be very neophobic, or suspicious of new foods. Sometimes these rejections are accompanied by disgust, the last emotion to show up in our developmental repertoire. It turns out that happiness arrives first, anger at about four months, and fear or surprise at six or seven months. We learn disgust through potty-training, and it's a welcome evolutionary step since disgust protects children from ingesting toxins as they become more mobile and start to explore the world, often

RAINBOW MEAL

Some dinners look as if you've drawn them with the vivid colors in a Crayola box. Here are a few variations on the theme of delicious, bright soups that can be combined with an open-faced sandwich to make a colorful meal. You can also freeze half of the soup and serve it the following week on a tired weekday night.

VEGETABLE SOUP

Precut vegetables such as squash, broccoli, cauliflower, or
    carrots, cut into 1- to 2-inch chunks
Potatoes, chunked (optional)
Apple or pear, peeled and chunked
Olive oil
1 onion, chopped
1 (16-ounce) carton chicken or vegetable stock
Salt and pepper to taste
1 tablespoon curry powder, or seasoning of your choice

Start by choosing a vegetable: squash (I recommend getting precut, so you don't have a slippery, hard-to-cut vegetable), broccoli, cauliflower, or carrots all work beautifully. Frozen spinach is also a winner (add it along with the stock). You can add potatoes to any of these choices, for extra hardiness.

Cut the vegetable (and optional potato) into chunks of about an inch or two and place on a lightly oiled cookie tray. Drizzle with olive oil, and then mix with clean hands so that all the chunks are fairly evenly coated with oil.

Place in preheated 400-degree oven for 30 to 50 minutes, depending on the hardness of the vegetables. When you have about 15 minutes to go, add the apple or pear, also coated lightly in olive oil.

While the vegetables are roasting, sauté the onion in olive oil in a soup pot or Dutch oven. When the onion becomes translucent, throw in the roasted vegetables and the fruit. Stir in the stock, and bring to a

boil, and let simmer for about 10 minutes to blend the flavors. Season
the soup with salt and pepper. I usually add curry powder but you
may want to experiment with other seasonings.

Let the soup cool a bit, and then puree in a food processor in small
batches until smooth (or leave it a bit choppy if you prefer a more
textured soup).

To accompany these dazzling soups, you can toast some bread and
spread with ripe avocado. Place some sliced cheese (Swiss and cheddar work well) on top of the avocado. Cook in a toaster oven until the
cheese melts over the avocado. For added color, you can sprinkle some
paprika on top. (These have been my go-to sandwiches for the last
forty years, and I never tire of them. I think I discovered them when
I lived on a commune in California, and I really don't know why they
haven't replaced peanut butter and jelly or tuna as classic sandwiches.)
Arrange a few pieces of fresh fruit on the plate and you will have a
veritable rainbow.

through their mouths.[12] It's a bit of a puzzle why some children are more
timid than others about trying new foods, and differences can vary within
a family, even when children and parents eat similarly. My sons, for example, love raw and cooked red meat, while I feel queasy at the very prospect
of these foods.

One answer to the question "Where does pickiness come from?" is
genes. A study of more than 5,000 pairs of twins, ages eight to eleven, found
that food pickiness was mainly inherited: 78 percent of food aversions were
reported to be genetic, while only 22 percent were attributable to environmental factors, such as the level of tension at the dinner table or the way
new foods are introduced or the quality of the cooking.[13] Perhaps, my sons'
taste buds were inherited from their father, who will try anything and finds
almost everything delicious.

Given that food pickiness is largely hard-wired, what can parents do
with the 22 percent that has to do with environmental factors? How can
parents encourage children to become more open to new foods?

Food pickiness tends to peak during toddlerhood. So try to introduce a variety of foods before that time, and try again when your child is older. Don't label your child as picky, as you might find that her taste buds become much more flexible during later childhood.

There are other strategies that can help. Children who participate in cooking meals are more likely to want to try their own creations. In a study at Columbia University, 600 kids in kindergarten through the sixth grade who took part in a cooking class were much more likely to eat the foods that they made than those who didn't take the class.[14]

Another strategy to promote adventurous eating is for parents to model their enjoyment of a broad range of foods. In one study, preschoolers tended to like or reject the same fruits and vegetables as their parents. "Oh, how I *love* these roasted Brussels sprouts" might inspire your little ones to get in on the action. Children of all ages will pick up on other food cues, too. Children of parents who talk about weight and dieting will be much more likely to use unhealthy weight-control strategies such as binging and purging. It's better to focus on healthy eating than on your concern about your child's weight.[15] And even more important than the talk is the parents' behavior: Those who are on diets are more likely to have kids with eating disorders.[16]

It's also important not to give up too soon. Many nutritionists offer the "rule of fifteen," or presenting the same food at least fifteen times to see if children will accept it.[17] The idea behind the rule of fifteen is that kids tend to like food that's familiar, so repeated exposure to a food will make it familiar. "Oh, this old snap pea; it's been around here a lot. I guess I might as well try it." A corollary here is to use foods that have gotten your child's stamp of approval to act as a bridge to new foods. For example, if your child wolfs down carrot sticks, you might introduce celery sticks, which have the same crunch, or sweet potatoes, which are similar in color. Or add a new vegetable into a stir-fry that contains some recognizable vegetables. Even if a child picks out the interloping broccoli florets, these new vegetables will become more and more familiar.

For most eaters, what we find repugnant in new foods is the texture. Tomatoes, mushrooms, and onions are the three most often rejected nonanimal foods.[18] If your child repeatedly rejects a food, you might try offering it in a new form with a different texture. You can sauté the mushrooms and onions first, and then puree them into a soup with trusted vegetables like carrots, which might render the slimy rascals more palatable.

Researchers at Duke's Center for Eating Disorders use relaxation techniques to help young children expand their food repertoires. While you might not want to chant "Om" at the table, a relaxed mood, conveyed by soft voices and restraint from critiquing a child's table manners, can go a long way to creating a calm atmosphere at the dinner table.

A counterintuitive piece of advice I've heard from pediatricians, which is also supported in the research literature, is for parents to refrain from rewarding kids for eating a particular food. It turns out that saying to your kids, "Eat your cauliflower and then you can have a piece of chocolate cake" will often backfire. What happens is that kids come to dislike foods they have been rewarded to eat.[19] And—a double whammy—their preference for the reward food increases.

Restricting such foods as cookies and potato chips is also a losing strategy. Researchers at Penn State University demonstrated that children want more of foods that are forbidden. Kids who were given unlimited access to cookie fruit bars ate fewer than those who were told they had to wait ten minutes. In fact, consumption of the restricted cookies *tripled* as compared to consumption of the freely available cookies. Those verboten cookies also elicited more positive comments than ones that were freely available.[20] Ever since the Garden of Eden, forbidden foods have been more attractive.

Offering a variety of fruits and vegetables to children is a great starting point, but it's not the whole story, because children aren't little bear cubs. They also need protein, dairy, fats, and grains. The U.S. Department of Agriculture (USDA) offers a helpful visual aid for balancing these different food groups—MyPlate.gov, which was unveiled in 2011 by Michelle Obama and Agriculture Secretary Tom Vilsack. The icon is a plate that is suggestive of proportions for a healthy diet:

- Make half your plate fruits and vegetables.
- Fill a quarter with a protein, such as lean meat, tofu, eggs, or fish, trying to vary your choices.
- Use the remaining quarter of your plate for grains, aiming for whole-grain choices for at least half of these.

• A small dairy recommendation is connoted in the shape of glass at the side of the plate.

At The Family Dinner Project, we recommend using the MyPlate programs' food list to help children brainstorm and broaden their food choices while also helping with the planning of meals. After explaining to kids how MyPlate works, invite them to choose foods from each of the five categories that they like, or think they might be willing to try. Then you can write down these choices on a downloaded icon of a plate and post it on the refrigerator for easy reference. Since kids' tastes are notoriously fickle, you will need to update the lists. In addition to helping with the cooking, identifying a variety of food choices is another way to get your kids involved in dinner making. An involved child is often a more engaged eater. Of course, you are the one ultimately in charge of making the choices and should use your own wider and deeper experiences to introduce foods that kids didn't put on their lists.

Michael Pollan also offers advice about healthy eating, positing that all you need to know is that there is no one diet that is preferable to any other, except for our current American diet, which is making us sick with processed food, meat, fat, sugar, and non–whole grains. He condenses his advice to a seven-word maxim: *Eat food. Not too much. Mostly plants.* This message, elaborated in his 2008 book, *In Defense of Food,* and in its more whimsical spin-off, *Food Rules,* is not quite as simple a set of dictates as those seven words would suggest. The command to "eat food" is about avoiding foods with ingredients you can't pronounce, foods that have sugar listed in the top three ingredients, foods that are sold in the middle aisles of the supermarket, and foods that won't rot. The injunction to "eat mostly plants" is aimed at encouraging eating mostly fruits and vegetables, and very little meat.

The command "not too much" flies in the face of how I grew up, when I was urged to "waste not, want not"—an admirable credo aimed at grateful frugality, and forged out of my parents' experiences with Depression-era scarcities. In many homes, children were told that they had to join the "clean plate club" before they could leave the table or get dessert. But with so many Americans overweight, and portion sizes ballooning, Pollan counters with the idea that it's better to stop eating when you're full, even if that means leaving food on your plate. In order to know when you've had enough, Pollan's last set of rules focuses on the context of eating—eat meals (rather than a series of snacks throughout the day) slowly so that you know when you are sated, eat with other people, and eat at a table (not in a car, in front of a TV, or at your computer).[21]

Ellyn Satter, a nutritionist and family therapist, and internationally recognized authority on eating and feeding, offers a very reasonable credo: "Feeding demands a division of responsibility. Parents are responsible for the what, when, and where of feeding; children are responsible for the how much and whether of eating." What follows from this philosophy is consistent with the research. Parents need to offer healthy, varied, attractive, appealing food, but they should not get caught up in cajoling, tricking, bargaining, or negotiating. Children need to learn to trust their own bodies to know when they're hungry and what they need to eat.

EMBRACE QUICK FOOD NOT FAST FOOD

Eating well requires some cooking. If you grew up with a parent who didn't cook, you might feel overwhelmed and clumsy in the kitchen. If you are a woman who feels that cooking has oppressed women for centuries, you might avoid the kitchen on principle. If you are already working one or two jobs, making a meal every night can feel like a bridge too far. And just

---

WHAT ARE "WHOLE GRAINS"?

Whole grains come in nutty, crunchy, interesting flavors like barley, quinoa, bulgur, faro, and brown rice. They can all be spruced up by tossing in some toasted nuts, scallions, herbs, or dried fruit. Sticking to whole-wheat breads can be a challenging project, as you have to read the labels carefully. As Marion Nestle suggests: "If you are looking for real whole-grain breads, look for 100 percent on the label, whole-wheat flour as the first ingredient, 2 grams of fiber per ounce."[22] If you can't go all the way with whole wheat, then second best is to look for breads with the fewest ingredients and without additives.

as some people hate to swim, or read, or watch football, you might hate to cook. I sympathize with each of these objections.

One remedy for the culinary-challenged and the time-challenged, and even those who just never warmed up to cooking at all, is to keep things simple and speedy in the kitchen. Forget about the twenty steps required to make Julia Child's fish quenelles, or making gefilte fish from scratch in the bathtub. Instead, focus on "fast food," which doesn't have to mean un-healthy, oversize meals with high fat and sugar content served in Styro-foam containers. That notion of fast food entered the Merriam-Webster dictionary in 1951, but fast food has actually been around for thousands of years. Ancient Romans grabbed a quick breakfast of bread soaked in wine from street vendors, and Europeans in the Middle Ages scarfed down pies and waffles sold on the street.

My mother, a feminist, believed in another version of fast food: She loved family dinners, but she hated to feel "stuck in the kitchen," so she got in and out as quickly as possible. Fast food in our home meant a meal that took less than half an hour, from fridge to stove to table. Heaven help you if you went in the kitchen while my mother was cooking. Fast food meant that she spun around in our small galley kitchen, grabbing vegetables with one hand, wrapping a potato in tin foil to throw in the oven with the other, and overseeing a chicken that spun itself on a rotisserie. She was a whirling dervish—her frantic pace left no room for help from family members until it was time to set the table and bring the food out. As for me, while I've al-ways admired my mother's efficiency in the kitchen, I prefer to bring others in to cook with me, so I don't feel stuck there alone.

I am a big fan of fast food when I think of it as quick-to-prepare food that is also inexpensive and healthy. I will call it "quick food." There are many strategies for creating quick, healthy, delicious dinners. Here are a few:

Have some "go to" meals that you can make from what is usually on hand

You'll obviously save time if you don't have to rush out to the store. Here are two of my go-to meals when I haven't planned ahead, don't feel like going out, and want something quick and nutritious.

FRITTATAS (FOR 4)

8 large eggs

¼ cup milk

Salt and pepper to taste

2 tablespoons oil or butter

3 cups vegetables (any combination of onions, asparagus, red pepper,
    scallion, cherry tomatoes, mushrooms, or whatever else you have
    on hand)

⅓ cup shredded Parmesan, cheddar, or Swiss cheese

Crack the eggs in a large bowl and whisk with milk, salt, and pepper.

In an all-metal skillet, heat the oil or butter, and then add the vegetables.
Sauté for 5 to 10 minutes, or until the vegetables are softened.

Pour the egg mixture over the vegetables, and let this concoction sit over
moderate heat until it looks mostly cooked through—less than 5 minutes.
Sprinkle the cheese over the egg mixture, and place the pan in the oven
under the broiler for about 5 minutes, or until it looks golden. When you
remove the pan from the oven be sure to use a pot holder.

Serve the frittata with a hunk of bread and a salad, and you'll have a
healthy, cheap meal made in less than 20 minutes.

BLACK BEAN BURGERS (FOR 4)

1 red bell pepper, chopped

2 carrots, minced

1 onion, chopped

2 garlic cloves, chopped

2 (15-ounce) cans black beans, rinsed and drained

2 large eggs

1 tablespoon cumin

1 tablespoon chili powder

1 cup breadcrumbs

Rolls or buns

STOCK CABINETS AND REFRIGERATOR
WITH FOODS TO HAVE ON HAND

Olive oil (for salads), canola oil for cooking, vinegars (balsamic, red-wine, white-wine), soy sauce

Mayonnaise, mustard

Fresh seasonings: whole onions and garlic

Dried seasonings: chili powder, cream of tartar, fennel seeds, cumin, curry powder, paprika, cayenne pepper, red chili flakes, kosher salt, table salt, pepper

Lemons and limes

Baking items: granulated sugar, brown sugar, honey, unsweetened cocoa powder, bittersweet or semisweet chocolate chips, whole-wheat flour, all-purpose flour, baking soda, baking powder

Canned goods: canned tomatoes, tomato paste, chicken broth, vegetable broth

Canned beans: chickpeas, black beans, red kidney beans

Pasta

Grains: barley, quinoa, bulgur

Breadcrumbs or panko

Nuts: walnuts, almonds, pine nuts, sesame seeds, pecans (keep in refrigerator to keep fresh)

Dairy: low-fat milk, hunk of Parmesan cheese, Swiss cheese, large eggs

Sauté the bell pepper, carrots, and onion in a small frying pan for about 10 minutes, or until the vegetables are soft. Add the garlic during the last few minutes (it needs less time than the other vegetables or it will get brown and bitter).

Mash the beans in a medium bowl by pressing down with a fork. In another bowl, whisk the eggs with the cumin and chili powder. Combine the vegetables, eggs, seasonings, and breadcrumbs with the beans, mixing into a sticky consistency. Form the mixture into four to six patties.

Sauté the patties in a skillet over moderate heat for 3 to 5 minutes on a side, flipping to brown on each side. Serve on toasted rolls or buns. (If I

have an avocado on hand, I mash it, and add salt, garlic, lemon, and a dash
of cayenne pepper. Then I put a dollop of this mixture on top of the black
bean burger.)

Use only one bowl, pot, or pan

This cuts down on the cleanup and tends to focus one's concentration. I
think it's also a time-saver not to have to keep referring to a recipe as you
proceed step by step. Instead, mix and match according to what is season-
ally available or with items floating around in your fridge. A good example
of this is the Meal-in-Bowl Salad.

MEAL-IN-BOWL SALAD

I haven't made a salad with carrots, cucumbers, and tomatoes in decades.
Why limit yourself when you can incorporate every food group and have a
complete meal? Here is a palette to choose from.

> **Pick a green:** arugula, Bibb lettuce, spinach, kale, dandelion greens.
> **Pick a fruit:** plum, peach, watermelon, grapes, pears, strawberries, rasp-
> berries, blood orange (my favorites).
> **Pick a vegetable (or more than one):** tomato, avocado, mushroom. Or
> use leftover roasted asparagus, broccoli, squash, or cauliflower.

A favorite variation on this salad is to choose a vegetable and fruit that
resemble each other in taste or appearance: a tomato and a plum; a cucumber and a grape; a peach and roasted squash.

> **Toast some nuts:** walnuts, pine nuts, almonds, and pecans. Toast them
> in a dry pan over low heat for about two minutes or until you start
> to smell the nut (toasting helps release the flavor).
> **Add some optional whimsy:** Parmesan chips (made by grating table-
> spoonfuls of Parmesan cheese that you bake on a baking sheet and in
> a 350-degree oven for about 7 minutes, or until golden brown). Or
> pick some edible flowers in the spring and summer seasons—violets,

dandelions, chive blossoms, bee balm, basil flowers, lavender, mint flowers, Johnny jump-ups, marigolds, or nasturtiums will all do the trick.

Make a dressing: Mix three parts oil (try walnut, hazelnut, olive) to one part vinegar (try balsamic, raspberry, strawberry). For extra flavor, whisk in a little mustard and any herbs that you like.

Pick a protein: grilled shrimp, leftover roast chicken, black beans, tofu, and kidney beans.

Top with cheese: Sprinkle or shave some Parmesan cheese on top.

My favorite combination is arugula, peaches, shrimp, avocados, and walnuts, with Parmesan chips. Another one I really like is spinach, plums, tomatoes, pine nuts, and chicken.

Make a meal that is easily repurposed into a second meal

You can get two meals from one trip to the supermarket by preparing a dinner that yields leftovers that can be the basis for tomorrow's dinner. A classic version of this is a roasted chicken with vegetables that gets transformed into a hearty chicken soup the following night. If you really want to save time, start with a rotisserie chicken picked up at the grocery store and skip the roasting instructions.

ROASTED CHICKEN

1 (3- to 4-pound) chicken
Vegetables, such as potatoes, fennel, carrots, squash, cut up
4 garlic cloves, unpeeled
Salt and pepper to taste
1 lemon or orange
Olive oil
Paprika

Preheat the oven to 400 degrees. Place a bunch of cut-up vegetables and garlic cloves in a large baking pan.

Rinse the chicken inside and out, removing any giblets, and pat dry with paper towels. Season the chicken with salt and pepper inside and outside. Stuff a lemon or orange (or half of each) into the cavity of the chicken. Drizzle oil over the chicken, using a brush to distribute evenly. Sprinkle with paprika if you want some nice color on your chicken. Place the chicken on top of the vegetables.

Bake in the oven for about 90 minutes. You'll know it's done when the leg wiggles easily and the juices run clear, not bloody. Remove the chicken from the oven and let it rest for about 20 minutes before serving.

CHICKEN SOUP

Leftover chicken
Chicken carcass
1 (16-ounce) carton chicken stock (optional)
2 carrots, peeled and chopped
1 stalk celery, chopped
1 large leek, cleaned and chopped
1 onion, chopped
2 cloves garlic
1 tablespoon olive oil
1 cup barley, rice, orzo, or quinoa
Diced parsley
Splash of lemon juice

For its second incarnation, remove the leftover chicken from the bones; dice the chicken and set aside. Remove and discard all skin. Place the carcass into 2 quarts of water. (I often cheat by adding a 16-ounce container of chicken stock because I don't have all day to boil the bones to make a fabulous stock.)

Sauté the carrots, celery, leeks, and onion in the oil in a medium frying pan until soft. Add the garlic and sauté for another minute. (Another time saver is to skip the sautéing and just throw the vegetables into the pot with the chicken.) Add the softened vegetables to the simmering stock.

TIPS FOR FREEZING

- Keep your freezer temperature at 0 degrees F or lower.
- Let foods cool down before freezing to prevent raising the temperature of your freezer and inducing uneven freezing.
- Portion foods into meal-size containers, making sure to label and date.
- When freezing liquids, allow for a small amount of breathing room at the top of the container, as liquids will expand when frozen.
- Be fierce about keeping extra air out of your packaging: Wrap meats and baked goods tightly in aluminum foil; use plastic containers with airtight lids for soups and stews.
- To defrost foods safely, move them from the freezer into the refrigerator, if you can plan ahead for this slow process. If not, you can defrost them by placing the frozen food in a leak-proof plastic bag that is then put into a large container of cold water. For speediest results, you can use the defrost setting on the microwave. However, don't use the microwave to defrost bread or rolls. You should wrap these in aluminum foil and bake in a preheated 425-degree oven for 3 to 5 minutes.

You could go an archaeological dig in my freezer, finding meat I froze before the iPhone was invented, and cakes that I didn't have the heart to throw out from parties given many years ago. While there is a school of thought that says freezing food preserves it for perpetuity, the flavor will eventually be affected. Here are some guidelines for "best if used by" for some common items:

Bread, muffins: 1 to 2 months

Baked fruit pies: up to 4 months

Cookie dough: up to 3 months

Soups and stews: 2 to 3 months

Meats: up to 1 year. (Note: Do not refreeze thawed meats. Once meat has thawed you need to cook it, and then it can be refrozen.)

Fish: up to 3 months

Cooked pastas: up to 2 months

Add the barley, rice, orzo, or quinoa; let simmer for 20 to 25 minutes. Remove the carcass. Add the shredded chicken, parsley, and lemon juice.

If your family starts to bellyache about leftovers, or if you make an excess of soup, don't forget your secret weapon—the freezer. Many dishes can easily be frozen for weeks or even months. Then when you pull them out again, voilà, they're no longer leftovers—it's as if you had a sous-chef doing the cooking for you while you were sleeping or practicing headstands.

Use a versatile cooking method that allows you to improvise with foods you have on hand

I'm particularly fond of creating different "schmears" to put on top of fish; then I bake or broil them in the oven. Bluefish, an aggressive and homely fish, is relatively inexpensive. It can be prepared quickly, and the results are very tasty.

BLUEFISH WITH SCHMEAR (FOR 4)

1½ pounds bluefish
1 tablespoon fennel seeds
⅓ cup mayonnaise
2 tablespoons mustard
1 garlic clove, minced
Canola oil

Rinse the bluefish and pat it dry. Roast the fennel seeds in a small dry pan for 2 minutes until they start to release an aroma; set aside.

For the schmear, combine the mayonnaise, mustard, garlic, and roasted fennel seeds in a small bowl.

Lightly oil a baking sheet, and place the fish on it, skin side down. Spread the schmear on the flesh side of the fish. Place the pan under the broiler for 15 to 20 minutes, or until the fish is flaky.

Other Schmears:

- In a food processor, mix 3 tablespoons butter, a handful of fresh basil, and a garlic clove. Smear this on a piece of fish that you bake in the oven at 375 degrees for about 15 minutes, adjusting for the thickness of the fish.
- Chop a blend of herbs, such as parsley, mint, and chives (about ⅓ cup each), and mix with 1 tablespoon Dijon mustard and juice from half of a lemon. Slowly add ¼ cup olive oil, until you have a nice paste for a topping. Wash and dry a piece of fish (about 1½ pounds of salmon, halibut, snapper, or haddock). Top the fish with the herb mixture and bake at 375 for 15 to 20 minutes, or until the fish is flakey.

Pasta is another food that allows for versatility in toppings. Since my children were toddlers, they have enjoyed a variety of pesto on pasta, with roasted chicken or grilled shrimp added in. Children as young as age three or four can help by pulling herb leaves off their stalks. The pesto recipe is simple.

PESTO

2 cups basil, parsley, watercress, or arugula (or a combination)
⅓ cup toasted pine nuts, walnuts, pecans, or almonds (or a
   combination)
¼ cup shredded Parmesan cheese
2 garlic cloves
Salt and pepper to taste
Olive oil

In a food processor, mix together all the ingredients except the olive oil. Blend into a thick paste. Slowly add olive oil until the pesto is a consistency that you like. Serve over pasta.

Customize dishes

Yet another strategy to help with healthy, fast, and delicious food—particularly when you have eaters who range from cautious to gourmand—

is the "customizing dish." Rather than turning yourself into a short-order cook, make one basic dish, and then let each member finish it to order. An extra bonus is that you can expose the cautious members of your family to other foods that they may venture to try next time.

My family's favorite version of this kind of eating is a Cambodian recipe, adapted from *The Elephant Walk Cookbook*. It's a basic chicken rice soup, or *jook,* to which each member adds what he or she wants; it's like making a sundae!

JOOK ADAPTATION (FOR 8)

4 chicken legs

2 cups jasmine rice

10 garlic cloves, divided

2 tablespoons vegetable oil, divided

3 tablespoons fish sauce (available in the Asian section of most
    supermarkets)

1 teaspoon sugar

1 teaspoon salt

½ pound mushrooms, carrots, red bell peppers, or a vegetable of
    your choosing (or a combination)

1 cup bean sprouts

1 lime, cut into wedges

1 bunch scallions, white parts, thinly sliced

Chili pepper flakes

Bring 2 quarts of salted water to a boil in a large pot. Add the chicken legs.

While the chicken is cooking, rinse the rice. Sauté two of the garlic cloves in 1 tablespoon of the oil in a large saucepan for 1 minute. Add the rice, stirring often, for about 5 minutes. When that's done, throw in with the chicken.

After the chicken has cooked for about 25 minutes, remove it and set aside, leaving the rice to continue cooking for about 15 minutes longer. Then add the fish sauce, sugar, and salt. Continue cooking for another 20 minutes. When the chicken cools, remove the skin, and pull the chicken off the bone, shredding it into bite-size pieces; add back to the soup.

Chop the remaining 8 cloves of garlic and sauté in the saucepan in the remaining tablespoon of oil for a minute or two, or until golden. Place the garlic in a small bowl.

Sauté the mushrooms, carrots, red pepper (or whatever combination you want) in the saucepan for a few minutes (add more oil if needed) or until tender; place them in another small bowl.

Place the bean sprouts, lime wedges, and scallions in individual bowls. Bring all the bowls to the table, along with the chili pepper flakes.

Serve each person the chicken rice soup. Let each person sprinkle in items of their choosing from the bowls.

I would be remiss not to confess that my ace in the hole is my husband. I cook like a cormorant spotting her prey for dinner: I focus straight ahead and never look back. In the process, I leave a trail of dirty dishes, onion peels, and vegetable detritus. My husband long ago took on the role of dishwasher, which he does in a mostly uncomplaining manner. Even when I do my own cleaning up, I hate to stop in the middle of cooking to tidy. I just like to go for it, even if that means I end up working on just the last few remaining inches of overcrowded counter space.

Any of these strategies is improved by having help and company in the kitchen. Like my mother, I don't like being stuck in the kitchen. But if my sons, husband, or a friend offer to chop the onions (a task I loathe), stir the risotto, or take over with me playing sous-chef, I don't care how long dinner takes to make. Then the focus is on creating something together and starting the dinner table conversation before we even sit down.

ILLNESSES, ALLERGIES, AND DEVELOPMENTAL DISORDERS THAT AFFECT EATING

It's hard enough to plan meals that everyone in your family will enjoy, but when one member has special dietary needs, the challenges multiply. Here are some considerations for a few problems—diabetes, autism, and food allergies—that might complicate eating. For each one, I offer some tips from experts about how to maintain a dinnertime ritual.

ACTIVITIES TO PROMOTE HEALTHY EATING

Do . . .

- Plant something edible on your windowsill—cherry tomato plant, basil, rosemary, chives.
- Create a colorful plate of food.
- Have a supermarket scavenger hunt (see box on page 71).
- Download MyPlate.gov.
- Stay on the perimeter of the supermarket, where the unprocessed foods are found.
- Take your kids to farmers' markets.
- Involve your children in cooking.
- Model your enjoyment of fruits and vegetables.
- Look through cookbooks with your kids.

Don't . . .

- Offer dessert as a reward for eating your vegetables.
- Give up on a food after offering it only a couple of times.
- Hide cookies and chips, or other forbidden foods.
- Take the kids to supermarkets unless you're prepared to wage a counteroffensive on marketing.
- Let your kids make all the decisions about food choices.
- Become a short order cook who makes as many different meals as there are people at the table.
- Diet in front of your children.
- Worry if your child isn't an adventurous eater.

When a family member has diabetes

There are two types of diabetes. **Type 1 diabetes** used to be called juvenile diabetes because it was the type of diabetes that most often affected children. Over the past few decades, however, a worldwide epidemic of childhood obesity has been accompanied by a dramatic increase in the incidence of Type 2 diabetes in children.

SUPERMARKET SCAVENGER HUNT

Is there any place more predictable than a supermarket for a child to have a tantrum? Who hasn't given in to buying Lunchables or a box of brightly colored cereal to stave off the public embarrassment of a meltdown? John Sarrouf and Grace Taylor at The Family Dinner Project came up with the idea of a supermarket scavenger hunt as a game to teach kids about food.

Give each child a list of items to find in the market. Some suggestions are: Find a fruit or vegetable of each color of the rainbow. Find one item that was grown or raised in your state. Compare the prices between a name-brand box of cereal and the store brand. Which is cheaper? Compare the grams of sugar in a nonfat flavored yogurt and a can of soda. Which has more? What foods are available at the checkout lines? Why? You can make up your own items and change them up according to the age of your child.

Type 2 diabetes, which used to be an illness that only occurred in adults, now accounts for 8 to 45 percent of new pediatric cases.[23] It is especially prevalent in low-income and minority populations, most likely because of the ease of accessing fatty, sugary fast foods and the difficulty of accessing healthy, fresh foods. With both types of diabetes, the intake of whole-grain carbohydrates (brown rice, whole barley, millet and wheat berries, whole-kernel bread) is recommended because these foods are digested slowly, which keeps blood sugar levels more even. Foods—such as white bread, pasta, soda, snack foods, canned fruits, cookies, and ice cream—which quickly turn food into sugar, should be avoided or minimized.[24] Other dietary recommendations are to eat lean protein at most meals, to eat nuts, and as many vegetables as desired. In other words, to a large degree, the diet for a diabetic is a healthy diet.

Ellen O'Donnell, a psychologist at Massachusetts General Hospital, works with kids who are having a hard time adjusting to a diabetes diagnosis. She knows this territory from the inside out because she was diagnosed with Type 1 diabetes when she was a senior in college. As she recalls, it was her parents that had the hardest time adjusting to the diagnosis. They tried to help Ellen by adapting their cooking into "diabetic" foods, but in the process many dishes were rendered inedible.

Ellen remembers her first Thanksgiving after the diabetes diagnosis. Her mother made her signature apple pie with Splenda. "It was terrible," she says. "I told them to make the foods the way you make them, and I'll just eat as much as I can." Her family also adjusted the timing of meals so that they were more regular. She had to eat within an hour of her injections.

Much has changed since Ellen was diagnosed about twenty years ago, when nutritional information was hard to find. She used to have to estimate her carbs. If she had a serving of rice the size of her palm, it was so many carbs. It was mostly trial and error. She would estimate how much insulin to take, and then check her blood levels, and adjust. She had to restrict her diet to foods for which she knew how much insulin to take.

Now she relies on several Smartphone apps, such as Epicurious, to figure out how many carbs are in a recipe so that she will know exactly how much insulin to give herself. She learned early on not to choose foods that were labeled low sugar, because she ended up substituting with fat. Instead, she shifted to looking for whole foods.

Now a mother of two young sons, Ellen says her family dinner is lively, if a bit complicated. Jonah, who is three, has a dairy intolerance—he gets puffy and bloated when he drinks milk or has cheese, yogurt, or ice cream. Her husband, Eric, has an allergy to tree nuts and is also lactose intolerant. Her son Luke, age nine, is the only family member without any food restrictions. Most nights, they try to eat the same basic meal but with lots of little modifications. When they have pasta, they get regular pasta and check the number of carbs, rather than buy the healthy pasta with chickpeas that her husband is allergic to. When they have pizza, Jonah has to have his without cheese. Only Ellen and Luke add nuts to their salads.

The kids have known about their mother's diabetes since they were preschoolers. Ellen recently overheard Jonah singing his own version of the hokey pokey: "Press your blood sugar in, press your blood sugar out." They understand that sometimes the family action has to pause so that their mother can eat. On a family outing, she might end up consuming all the snacks so as to prevent the plummeting of her blood sugar. And when the boys see their mother's hands shaking because of low blood sugar, one of them will ask if she needs a banana.

When I asked Ellen what advice she had for families when a member has diabetes, she used a cooking analogy. "Diabetes should always be on the back burner," she says. "If you're cooking pasta and making sauce, the sauce is on the front burner and you need to pay attention to it so it doesn't splatter. The sauce is the most important part of the dinner because it provides the flavor. The diabetes is like the pasta—well controlled enough so that it's not boiling over. But it should be on the back burner. You want it be under good enough control so that you can focus on the other things that are more important."

She tells me another lesson, using her mother's apple pie to illustrate. If you are eating well during the week, there is no reason not to have a piece of pie on the weekend. Rather than having the diabetic version of apple pie, with a sugar substitute, she says "it's better to have the pie that I want rather than make it all about diabetes."

When a child has autism spectrum disorder

Autism spectrum disorder (ASD) is a group of developmental brain disorders characterized by impairment in communication and social interaction, as well as by repetitive behaviors such as rocking, and by obsessive interests in a particular subject like vacuum cleaners, numbers, or elephants. It affects an estimated one in sixty-eight children.[25] ASD often permeates eating— even past the age when most kids outgrow food pickiness, kids with ASD continue to be selective eaters. They can be very sensitive to the texture of foods, accepting only crunchy foods or pureed ones, or they may have idiosyncratic eating behaviors, such as only drinking from a sippy cup.

Stephen Shore, the author of a memoir about having autism, wrote this vivid description of his relationship with food: "Canned asparagus was intolerable due to its slimy texture, and I didn't eat tomatoes for a year after a cherry tomato had burst in my mouth while I was eating it. The sensory stimulation of having that small piece of fruit explode in my mouth was too much to bear, and I was not going to take any chance of that happening again."[26]

Carol Singer, Ph.D., is a child psychologist in the Boston area who specializes in working with kids on the autism spectrum. She explains that there are several ways that family meals can be challenging for kids on the spectrum, particularly when any changes in the routine create anxiety. A holiday dinner with added guests, a change in the timing of dinner, or even the introduction of new foods can be changes that are upsetting to children with ASD.

When kids feel anxious Dr. Singer teaches them skills to practice at the dinner table or while taking a break from dinner. One is to develop a hand signal that a child can use when he is feeling overwhelmed or can't stay at the table. Learning to use a hand signal is far preferable to waiting until the child is so upset that he becomes disruptive. In addition, Singer suggests that when children are anxious that they play "Freeze-Melt"—the child is told to tighten all his muscles and "freeze" for a moment, and then relax all over. Or a child can practice "mindfulness" by describing an object without judging how she feels. Does the object feel heavy, cold, soft? These skills could be helpful for any child (or adult) to practice when feeling overwhelmed by an interaction at the table.

Kids with autism often are very sensitive to noise, which can make it hard for them to sit through a dinner when several people are talking at the same time. If it's a holiday dinner, with many more voices at the table, the child with ASD can find it hard to keep up because of disturbances in his auditory processing. This difficulty might quickly translate to feeling anxious, which will, in turn, make it more difficult to participate at the table.

The sensitivities that often accompany ASD can interrupt dinner in another way. Sam, an eight-year-old boy whom Dr. Singer saw in therapy, developed an exquisite aversion to hearing his sister, Dahlia, clear her throat.[27] This aversion had begun when Sam awoke in the middle of the night to find red lights flashing and sirens blaring. His sister was having an asthma attack and needed emergency intervention. Afterward, whenever Sam heard his sister clear her throat, he was terrified that she would have an asthma attack. And Sam was afraid that if he was around someone clearing his throat, he could catch it and give it to his sister. Unfortunately, Dahlia often cleared her throat at the dinner table, and Sam would go flying away from the table when she did.

Dr. Singer used exposure therapy to restore the dinner hour. First she wrote the letters "TC" for throat clearing, and then spelled it, and then she said it. Once, Sam could bear these exposures to throat clearing, Dr. Singer recorded the sound of throat clearing off the Internet, then recorded her own voice making the noise. Then Dahlia recorded herself clearing her throat. Finally, Sam was asked to stay at the table three nights a week while Dahlia made the noise. With the process of gradually acclimating himself to the sound, Sam learned to tolerate it.

As with any disability affecting a child, siblings need to adapt and respond. If a child with ASD is allowed to eat pasta at every meal while his siblings must eat a healthier diet, or if he is allowed to leave the table to watch TV when the others must stay until dinner is over, it might feel unfair to the other children.

A child with ASD usually has many fewer peer contacts than her siblings and wants to spend more time with her siblings than vice versa. The parent might require the children without ASD to be home for dinner as much as possible, to provide modeling and companionship, but those children can be chafing to spend more time out of the house with friends. The parent will likely feel torn between the different needs of her children.

When a child has a food allergy

The number of kids with food allergies—when the immune system goes into overdrive in response to substances usually considered harmless—increased from 3.4 percent in 1998 to 5.1 percent in 2011, according to the National Center for Health Statistics.[28] These kids' bodies release too much of an antibody, immunoglobulin E, in order to fight off the food allergens. As a result, the body releases histamine and other chemicals, which can make it hard to breathe, and hard for the blood to circulate. Epinephrine will halt a life-threatening reaction to a food allergy, but a better strategy is to avoid contact with the offending food. The most common allergies—peanuts, tree nuts, milk, eggs, wheat, soy, fish, and shellfish—account for 90 percent of allergic reactions.

Jen Haugen, RD, LD, works as a registered dietician in a supermarket, Hy-Vee, in Rochester, Minnesota, teaching healthy eating in one of the best classrooms—the grocery store aisles. While at the supermarket, she urges parents to read labels carefully, using a food allergy list that's updated yearly and covers the eight major allergens.[29] She also recommends serving the same meal to all family members by making small adjustments to accommodate a food allergy. For example, soymilk is a good substitute for cow's milk when a child is lactose intolerant, sunflower butter can be exchanged for peanut butter when there is a peanut allergy, and gluten-free bread works well for someone with celiac disease.[30]

Maintaining a sense of normalcy around healthy eating should be balanced by a suitable dose of vigilance. If an allergy is life threatening, that food should be banned from the house because the risk of an accidental ingestion is too high. And cooks should be mindful of the dangers of "cross contact,"—utensils, dishes, and cutting boards cannot be used for both verboten and permissible foods. A knife that has been dipped into the peanut butter jar should never be the same one used to spread jelly for a child with a peanut allergy. While food allergies are usually lifelong, there are some studies afoot to see if adults with allergies can become desensitized to lose them. My friend Tristan is ingesting a few milligrams of peanut powder each week, increasing the amount gradually, so that in two years he expects to be able to eat two Reese's peanut butter cups. No one, however, should attempt to overcome an allergy without the advice of a medical professional.

All of these conditions require extra planning, flexibility, and resourcefulness on the part of the cooks and fellow diners. Regardless of the eating challenges, preferences, or idiosyncrasies of individual family members, the goal of preparing food is the same—to bring family and friends together to the table. The food creates the occasion for dinner, but dinner is about so much more than the food.

We turn now to the additional elements of dinner that transforms it from a time to eat to a time to play and have fun.

5

Play with Your Food

The suggestion that you and your children play with food may seem a bit subversive, or just plain messy. I certainly grew up being told not to play with mine, especially when I built my peas into a pyramid or pushed around the gristly meat parts to disguise the fact that I wasn't eating everything on my plate. Later, as a mother myself, I wasn't amused when my son confessed that he had earned a weeklong detention for his role in a middle school cafeteria food fight. And I used to flee the kitchen when my husband commandeered our sons to help put away the groceries by "playing catch" with cans and bags hurled across the kitchen.

But maybe my husband was on to something. The kitchen is the heart of the home, the place where most of us gravitate. So why not make it a play station for creative projects, as well as a workstation for preparing meals? As we spend more time in virtual realms, the opportunity to make things with our hands becomes more precious.

Food, in its rainbow of colors and its range of textures from slippery oils to squishy pretzel dough, is a medium like paint or clay. Each of the different properties of food—size, shape, taste, smell, color—can become a focus of pleasurable investigation. And the very process of cooking lends itself to the scientific process of experimentation, since you can change one flavor or ingredient at a time, and keep testing the impact. The processes of transfor-mation in cooking, like adding fire or air, bring immediate and dramatic results, empowering the young creator with the feeling of "look what I can make!" The context in which food is eaten is also malleable and open to fooling around with—what music you listen to while you cook and where you eat are all elements at play.

Here are a few play episodes that have transpired in kitchens and din-ing rooms, summer camps and beaches, in my family, as well as the fam-ilies of my patients, students, and friends. Perhaps they will inspire you and your children to try new foods, and to linger longer in the kitchen for conversation.

PLAY WITH COLOR

One of my earliest memories is of my mother drawing a face on the shell of a soft-boiled egg resting in an eggcup. With a quick few flourishes of a magic marker, she would make curly hair tumbling out of a sun hat. Then with a serrated knife she'd cut around the top of the egg, so its "hat" could be removed. The rest of the egg might be a mustachioed man with glasses or a girl with a shy smile like mine. She'd present the egg with its "hat" on so that I could remove it and scoop out the insides. I never warmed up to the sliminess of a soft-boiled egg, but I loved to see what my mother would draw for me, so I would take a few bites to make sure she didn't give up on this activity.

Over the years, I've engaged my sons in activities that involve food for collage or painting. As Marcella Hazan, the Italian cookbook writer, put it, "Cooking is an art, but you eat it too."

It's fun to take the elements of a salad—sliced red pepper, cucumbers, avocado, carrot sticks, lettuce leaves, cherry tomatoes, bean sprouts, and nuts—and have each person make a face out of these elements on a plate. A cherry tomato placed on top of a cucumber slice makes a compelling eye-ball, and an avocado slice curves to make an elegant eyebrow. Lettuce and bean sprouts lend themselves nicely to hair and beards. Once you've had enough with faces, you can move on to making animals, cars, boats, planes, and houses. For hygiene purposes, it's a good idea to have each artist eat his or her own creation. If you need ideas and inspiration, do a Google "images" search for Giuseppe Arcimboldo.

Even more popular than making these collages was decorating cookies. When I ask my twenty-something sons about their favorite childhood memories, baking cookies as a family is near the top of their lists. Over the years, we have collected many recipes for holiday cookies, but this one, from my mother-in-law, is the best. These cookies make excellent holiday gifts or can serve as a centerpiece for a party at any time of the year. Confronted with a platter of these colorful cookies, guests alternate between thinking they look too good to eat and diving right in to bite off a chocolate head.

SUGAR COOKIES

(From my mother-in-law, Mary Daly)

⅔ cup unsalted butter
¾ cup sugar
½ teaspoon vanilla
½ teaspoon grated orange peel
1 large egg
4 teaspoons milk
2 cups all-purpose flour
1½ teaspoons baking powder
¼ teaspoon salt
Glaze (recipe follows)

In a mixer, thoroughly cream the butter, sugar, vanilla, and orange peel. Add the egg and beat until the mixture is light and fluffy. Then stir in the milk.

In a separate bowl sift together the flour, baking powder, and salt. Then stir the dry ingredients into the creamed mixture, blending well.

Divide the dough into two dough balls. Put each ball of dough in a piece of floured wax paper and store in the refrigerator for at least an hour (it can be kept for weeks).

When you're ready to make cookies, remove one dough ball from the refrigerator, warm it briefly in your hands until it is pliable, and then place it on a floured counter. Roll it out so the dough is about ⅛ inch thick. Cut with cookie cutters. (Some of our favorites are reindeer, dogs that look like our golden retriever, Christmas trees, dreidels, stars, musical notes, moons, dog bones, mother, father, and children shapes.)

Bake the cookies on a lightly greased cookie sheet in a 375-degree oven for about 8 minutes. (Watch them so they don't burn; oven temperature and the thickness of your dough sometimes vary, which might mean quicker doneness). Cool and decorate with glaze.

Glaze:

Powdered sugar

Milk

Food coloring

Make up several small ramekins with different colors. For each ramekin, combine ½ cup powdered sugar, a drop or two of milk, and a drop of food coloring. Mix very slowly, adding liquid to the sugar until you get a consistency that will spread smoothly on a cookie without running off.

You can also melt chocolate to decorate such things as the base of the tree, the fur of the dog, the horns on the reindeer, or the pants of the father. Some cookies may look like Jackson Pollock stopped by to add a colorful splatter, while others will have the careful, folk-art approach more suggestive of a visit from Grandma Moses.

As long as you have the food coloring out, you might want to try food coloring paintings. When my sons were young, I used to assemble two eye-droppers, several small dishes filled with water, different food colorings, and a pile of paper towels. They folded the paper towels into squares, or kept folding them into a tight pile, and applied drops of different colors. When the towels were unfolded, the patterns surprised and delighted us. We hung them up to dry on clotheslines strung around the kitchen. It was like stepping into a psychedelic Rorschach.

My colleague Dr. Mai Uchida grew up in Japan before coming to Boston for psychiatry training. On top of her demanding call schedule, patients, and supervision, she somehow also managed to take courses in fashion, and indeed she has a color sense to die for. She told me that she began developing this color sense at her grandmother's dinner table in Tokyo.

When Mai was a young child, her grandmother used to instruct her: "Eat your food as if you are painting a picture in your stomach." The idea was to picture each food as a paint color. She imagined the reds from a tomato as roses in her stomach, the brown of the rice filling in the soil for those roses, and the yellow from egg yolks getting transformed into butterflies swooping around the roses. In no time, the meal had translated into a painting, and in the process, Mai had been encouraged to eat a healthy rainbow of colors. Once she was old enough, Mai wanted to make the creations in the real world, not just in her stomach. One such creation is a birthday cake made out of sushi ingredients (see Sushi Birthday Cake recipe).

You can try "stomach-painting" at your table: Ask family members to share images of what each color of their food might paint in their stomach. Perhaps, like Mai, your kids will want to draw, sew, or cook the images that were inspired by their dinners.

SUSHI BIRTHDAY CAKE (FOR 6)

Cake:

  1½ cups brown rice
  1½ cups white rice
  3 cups cold water, divided
  4 tablespoons rice vinegar
  3 tablespoons sugar
  1 teaspoon salt
  4 tablespoons rice vinegar
  3 tablespoons granulated sugar
  1 teaspoon salt

Filling:

  1 (5-ounce) package dried seaweed, thinly sliced
  About 8 ounces of sushi- or sashimi-grade tuna or salmon

Topping:

  2 large eggs, scrambled with a splash of soy sauce
  ½ cup chopped green beans
  Pickled thin slices of carrots and bamboo shoots

Directions:

For the cake, rinse the rices, one type at a time, with cold water. When the water runs mostly clear of starch, drain the rice. Cook each rice type in a medium saucepan with 1½ cups cold water. Cook on high heat until the rice comes to a boil. Reduce the heat to simmer and cover with a lid. Let cook for 15 minutes, turn off the heat, and let the rice steam for 10 more minutes.

While the rice is cooking, combine the rice vinegar, sugar, and salt in a small bowl. Spoon the brown rice into one bowl and the white rice into another. Pour half of the vinegar mixture over each bowl while the rice is hot. Gently combine the rice and vinegar using a side-to-side cutting motion with a wooden spoon. The rice should be fluffy and shiny, warm but not hot. On a large plate spread a layer of brown rice, then seaweed, then white rice, then tuna, continuing the layering until all ingredients are used.

Decorate with the eggs, green beans, carrots, and bamboo shoots.

PLAY WITH SHAPE

Doughs of many kinds can be plied and twisted into recognizable shapes, and it's fun for kids to get their hands goopy and sticky. While bread usually requires patience to wait for rising, pretzels provide much quicker gratification. As an extra bonus, when eaten hot out of the oven, they evoke the pretzels sold from pushcarts in New York City's Central Park. In your own kitchen, kids can go wild molding the dough into different shapes.

PRETZELS

1½ cups warm water

1 (¼-ounce) package yeast

1 teaspoon table salt

1 tablespoon sugar

4 cups all-purpose flour

1 large egg, beaten with a little water

Kosher salt for sprinkling

Pour the warm water into a large mixing bowl. Sprinkle on the yeast and stir. Add the table salt, sugar, and flour. Mix and knead the dough.

Give each child a small ball of dough to roll and twist into letters, numbers, animals, or shapes without names. Grease a cookie sheet and place the pretzels on the sheet. Brush the pretzels with the beaten egg and sprinkle with kosher salt. Bake at 425 degrees for 12 to 15 minutes. Cool slightly before you plunge into these hot doughy delights.

PLAY WITH SIZE

I think that children's awareness of their own smallness creates an affinity for other small things, such as puppies, stuffed animals, and miniature figures. Playing with the size of foods, much as Alice played with her own height in *Alice in Wonderland,* seems to appeal to many children. Just cutting sandwiches into minis can be a treat, so long as they aren't the kind of sandwiches that ooze and drip with each cutting. Melted cheese, cream cheese with smoked salmon or sliced cucumber, or peanut butter with banana all lend themselves to bite-size sandwiches. These could be accompanied by mini-pops made by pouring juice into an ice tray and sticking a toothpick into each cube before putting the tray into the freezer. Kids may also be more willing to try a new food in a mini size that they wouldn't otherwise taste.

Experimenting with giant foods is also fun. You can take a chocolate chip recipe and bake most of it into one giant cookie in a pizza pan.

PLAY WITH TASTE

There are five flavors that our tongues can taste—sweet, sour, salt, bitter, and umami. Sweet, salt, and sour are easily identifiable and make for straightforward pairings of flavor with food: Sweet ice cream, salty pretzels, and sour lemons are some obvious combinations. Bitter is a paradoxical taste because it can serve as a warning that we are about to consume a toxic substance or it can be the signature taste of some very popular foods and drinks. Beer, coffee, olives, and marmalade all rely on bitterness to make their statement.

The least familiar to most eaters will be umami, a Japanese word meaning delicious. It's the new kid on the block. The two taste receptors for umami were identified as recently as 2000 and proved that the tongue has a special place on it to register the scrumptiousness of foods like steak, mushrooms, soy sauce, meat stocks, and Parmesan cheese.[1] Often an umami element unlocks a flavor burst from another food, as when we dip sushi into soy sauce, make risotto with a complex veal stock, or sprinkle Parmesan cheese on tomatoes.

Just as you might urge your kids to eat a wide variety of colors, you might also encourage tasting across the five different flavors, not only because there are obvious health benefits but also to boost experimentation with new foods. One way to do this is to ask your kids to think up a menu that uses all five tastes and then try to make it. For example, you could make pasta with roasted vegetables (salted), adding a sprinkle of Parmesan (umami). As an appetizer, whip up an olive (bitter) tapenade by mixing olive, capers, lemon juice (sour), garlic, and olive oil in a food processor and then spread on crackers. Baking cookies for dessert would give you your fifth taste sensation—sweet.

Another way to play with taste is to combine different foods in unexpected ways and ask your children to guess which taste buds are being activated. Try putting salt on a peach, or sugar on a piece of fish, or a squeeze of lemon on a potato.

Can you think of any dish that combines three flavors on your tongue? Salted coffee ice cream is one. How about four or five flavors? Roasted salted chicken with olives, lemons, and oranges. I'm sure you can think of many more.

But simplest of all is to ask your diners to guess the ingredients in a new dish. Sometimes, I like to throw an offbeat spice or flavor element into a meal to see if I can stump my family—a dash of cinnamon, a splash of lime juice, or a squirt of fish sauce can enhance the flavor of a dish while staying under the radar of taste detection. Don't be surprised if the children at the table are better at this game than the adults, since we lose half of our taste buds by age twenty.

PLAY WITH SMELL

The pleasures of taste rely on the aroma of food. In fact, the perception of flavor is dominated by smell, not by what our taste buds can detect. Scientists have recently discovered that humans can detect a trillion odors, but each person's preferences for and sensitivities to certain smells vary widely from individual to individual.[2] No wonder that the smell of blue cheese is heavenly to one person and smells like dirty socks to another, or that the smell of roasted coffee can be divine or nauseating. Did you know that only about 22 percent of the population has the genes to smell the rotten egg smell in urine that results from eating asparagus?

When I was growing up, one of my favorite birthday party activities was a smell test. Small jars with cinnamon, mint, toothpaste, bananas, or whatever was lying around would be lined up. The partygoers would wear a blindfold and take turns guessing what they smelled. Whoever got the most correct guesses got a prize. Years later, I used to play a version of this game with my sons, skipping the prize. I'd have them close their eyes and try to guess the smells I'd laid out on the kitchen table. It was a source of consternation when one boy could smell something as clearly as hearing a train whistle and the other boy smelled nothing.

Dr. Robin Schoenthaler, a radiation oncologist at Massachusetts General Hospital, writes about playing another variation of this game with her children as a way to make them more adventurous eaters. Every few months, she took her children to a local spice store, Penzeys, and let them smell as many spices as they wished. Then each child was allowed to buy one spice jar and use it on any dish they wanted until the spice ran out. "This way, their palate expanded just a bit," she explained.[3]

PLAY WITH FIRE

Fire, in all its uses, has always captivated the human mind. Perhaps cooking over an open fire evokes fantasies about being Robinson Crusoe stranded on a deserted island, or it rekindles memories of singing songs around a campfire during your first summer away from home. Fire even conjures the evolutionary argument that cooking with fire makes us human, since cooking with heat frees up the tremendous energy required to chew raw food, thus allowing humans to pursue activities other than digestion.[4]

There is something thrilling about cooking over an open fire at the beach. It's magical to be there at sunset when everyone else has gone home and the fireflies sparkle in the marshes and the stars begin to twinkle up above. With a little forethought you can take along some sticks, newspaper, and matches to get the whole thing started and then comb the beach for driftwood. Scoop out a shallow hole and form a ring of stones around it—this will make a good resting spot for the wood. Once the fire is under way, you can toast marshmallows on a stick and eat them as special gooey treats, or make s'mores by creating a sandwich of graham crackers with chocolate bars and toasted marshmallows in the middle.

Recently I made banana boats, a variation on the campfire classic. You'll want to assemble these before going to the beach.

BANANA BOATS (EACH PACKET SERVES 1 PERSON)

1 banana
4 squares chocolate
3 marshmallows

Slice each banana down the middle (keeping the skin on, and keeping the banana whole). Alternate placing pieces of chocolate and marshmallows in the cavity with the banana. Wrap the stuffed banana tightly in aluminum foil.

When ready to enjoy the treats at the beach, toss the packets in the embers for 5 to 10 minutes A bit of heaven will ensue: a hot, luscious confection that must be eaten with a spoon.

PLAY WITH AIR

If you like the idea of creating something out of nothing, then you'll enjoy these recipes. Breathtaking in its simplicity, but fun for kids and grownups, is to place whipping cream in a tightly covered Tupperware container. (Test the tightness of the lid first, to prevent wardrobe disasters.) Then just shake the daylights out of it. You can put on music and dance with it. Pass it from person to person and do the hokey pokey. After a few minutes, thanks to the addition of air, the cream will thicken to become whipped cream.

When The Family Dinner Project hosts community dinners, kids go off with one team member to shake up some whipped cream, and then put dollops of it on a berry crisp. This activity frees up enough time for the parents to talk and share strategies for overcoming common challenges to making dinner.

While the whipped cream recipe is fun and dramatic, if I had to pick my favorite recipe, it would be my meringue cookies, the recipe that feels like fashioning something delicious out of thin air. As an added bonus, these cookies are so quick to make that it takes less time to bake them than it does to drive to the store and buy a box of cookies. This recipe makes about twenty cookies. They don't keep that well, but then you probably won't have any left over. One caveat: You can't make them on a humid or rainy day. The egg whites just won't whip into shape.

MERINGUE COOKIES (MAKES ABOUT 20)

2 large egg whites

⅛ teaspoon salt

⅛ teaspoon cream of tartar

1 teaspoon vanilla

¾ cup sugar

6 ounces chocolate chips

⅓ cup toasted and chopped almonds, walnuts, or pecans (optional)

2 sheets of computer paper or parchment paper

Preheat the oven to 300 degrees. Whip the egg whites, salt, cream of tartar, and vanilla in a mixer until soft peaks form. Slowly add the sugar, while the machine is still running. The mixture should form peaks. Fold in the chocolate chips and toasted nuts.

Place the computer or parchment paper on the cookie pan. Using a tablespoon, spoon a rounded mound of the batter onto a cookie pan.

Place the cookies in the oven for about 25 minutes, or until they are lightly golden. If you just can't wait, you can take the cookies out at this point and they will be delicious, with a marshmallowy consistency. Better still: Turn off the oven after they cook for 25 minutes, and let them sit in the cooling oven for another hour. Then they will form a slightly crisp exterior with a pillowy interior. Because they are so airy, people eat them with abandon.

PLAY WITH LANGUAGE

Have you ever noticed how many foods are introduced in children's books? There are magical noodles in *Strega Nona,* the pomegranates that lure Persephone into Hades, and the irresistible Turkish delight in *The Lion, the Witch and the Wardrobe*. Then there is the treat created by drizzling maple syrup on snow in *Little House in the Big Woods,* and the delightful tribute to picky eaters, *Green Eggs and Ham*. Let's not forget *The Very Hungry Caterpillar,* who eats a feast before he turns into a butterfly, or the mouse that is given a cookie and has many adventures before finally getting a glass of milk. This doesn't even include the myriad of children's poems and nursery rhymes that involve, to name a few, porridge, blackbird pie, rice pudding, and strawberry jam. There is also the linguistic affinity between words and eating, as evidenced by language that bridges the two—eating your words, devouring a good book, thirst for knowledge, food for thought.

It can be fun to combine the worlds of eating and reading by creating foods or meals from favorite books. What might Harry Potter's quidditch stew be composed of? What about creating a high tea that is described in *Mary Poppins*? Or perhaps toast some bread with jam and then read *Bread and Jam for Frances* aloud at the table?

One of my friends belongs to a book group where, in addition to discussing the book, they also make food to accompany their discussions. The foods are chosen by virtue of having been mentioned in the book, or because they come from the country where the book takes place. This practice could translate to the reading of children's books as well—kids' appetites for discussing a book might be whetted by eating a food that plays a role in the book.

Food Poems

For younger kids, I turn to inspiration from my friend Lisa Price, who makes up food poems with her six-year old twins, a son and a daughter, an activity that helps them slow down and pay attention to what is going on in the moment. She discovered the power of poetry one evening when all her other efforts had failed to settle down her giggling, joking, squirming young children. She recalled that she wanted to pull out a bit of magic and drama.

"What if I told them that something amazing was right in front of them?" she wondered. As a bit of performance art, she paused, took a breath, was visibly awed by what she was looking at (a strawberry, as it turned out), and slowly uttered a short haiku-like poem: "Soft pillows, furry on my tongue. Tart. Smiling." Her children giggled and wanted to participate. She urged them to think about the color, the smell, the taste, the season of a food they were eating. How does it feel on your tongue, in your tummy? What mood are you in after tasting it? She also encouraged her kids to draw connections across time and space. For example, she asked them: "Does the warm potato on your plate remind you of the farm stand where we found it or the toasty blanket around your feet at last night's fire?" Taking turns, they each offered up a short poem. Her son's offering: "Kumquats surprise me. Make me have a face." When it was her daughter's turn, she said, "Tomatoes taste good when I eat them. Tomatoes spray inside my mouth!"

PLAY WITH MEMORY

Perhaps food is overrepresented in our memory banks because the experience of eating is simultaneously encoded in different parts of the brain—taste, color, texture, sound, and smell receptors all have a chance to build synapses. This multisensory experience of eating creates vivid memories. I think this partly explains why we remember holiday meals so clearly—because the sensory experience is heightened with music, wearing special clothes, and eating particularly aromatic foods. The more the senses are stimulated during an event, the greater the chance that we will remember that experience. We also tend to remember experiences and facts when there is a story connected to them. Since many memorable stories are told at the table, by and about the people who matter the most to us, we tend to hold on to them. The meals that accompany those stories also get stored in our memory banks.

There is a subgenre of literary works devoted to memoirs that revolve around food. Ruth Reichl's *Comfort Me with Apples,* Gabrielle Hamilton's *Blood, Bones and Butter,* Kate Christenson's *Blue Plate Special,* Gus Samuelsson's *Yes Chef,* and Laurie Colwin's *Home Cooking* are some of my favorite books that also happen to be food memoirs.

But you don't have to be a memoirist to play with your own childhood food memories. When you think back to your childhood days, are there certain foods that you really loved to eat? Was there a special side dish that showed up just for a holiday dinner? Did your grandparents or other elders make a dish that you remember fondly or that makes you hungry to think about now? Are there any meals you had that have a story that went with them? Perhaps there were kitchen disasters, food poisonings, or plates of delicious cookies that the dog ate and almost died from.

Were there any desserts that still make you salivate? Are there any foods that you closely associate with a beloved family member, so that when you eat that food, you think about him or her and feel moved to tell a story? If so, making that food for your family may be a way to bring that person to the table, if only in spirit.

For me, one such recipe is my mother's ice-cream cake. My mother was an artist whose favorite medium was clay. She made Hanukkah menorahs that looked like street scenes, lamps that were constructed with multiple coils to be castles, and boxes in the shapes of animals and beds. When it came to cooking, she favored dishes that were quick, but she wasn't afraid to muck around with food as though it were a piece of clay. I loved to help her make a particular cake that she made for every dinner party she ever hosted. Those parties were elegant affairs, with place cards and tablecloths, a caviar egg pie served as an appetizer, and our best silver trotted out for the night.

Her ice cream cake, made in about 10 minutes, was the capstone for her parties. My sister and I tried to stay up late enough to get a piece after the guests had been served. But, the next day, with the heavy cream hardened on the cake, it was even better.

Years later, my son Gabe always asked for ice cream cake for his mid-winter birthday. One year, I decided to make my mother's ice cream cake, and I even jazzed it up a bit by pouring hot fudge sauce on top. Alas, he told me that although it was delicious, he would prefer that I get him the ice cream cake that he was used to—from the Carvel store.

MY MOTHER'S (EDITH FISHEL) ICE CREAM CAKE

Cake:

About 2 dozen ladyfingers

3 pints ice cream, softened but not melting (my mother usually used mint chocolate chip, black raspberry, and chocolate because she thought these looked beautiful together).

Topping:

½ pint heavy cream

Colored sprinkles (optional)

Directions:

Line the bottom of a springform pan with ladyfingers (soft, yellow spongy cakes that are about 3 inches long and an inch wide). Then prop a ring of ladyfingers around the perimeter of the pan so that they are standing up and so that no part of the pan is showing.

Spoon out the first pint of ice cream and press it down, using a spatula or the palm of your hand. Then do the same with the next flavor of ice cream, and the next. Put the cake into the freezer. Just before serving, and as you let the cake warm up a bit, whip the heavy cream by hand with a beater or in an electric mixer until peaks form; be careful not to let the cream go too far and turn into butter. Spoon this whipped cream over the top of the cake before serving. (My mother used to decorate the cake with edible silver balls, which I think may be a bit toxic, so I skip them. Instead, colored sprinkles look nice on top.)

At the risk of gilding the lily, I like to serve the cake with Hot Chocolate Sauce drizzled over each beautiful slice.

HOT CHOCOLATE SAUCE

8 ounces quality chocolate

½ cup heavy cream

1 tablespoon honey

1 tablespoon freshly made coffee

Melt the chocolate and the cream in the top pan of a double boiler. Remove from heat and stir in the honey and the coffee.

PLAY WITH SPACE

Ask not only "what to have for dinner" but also "where to have dinner." Changes in context often alter the mood of dinner. Consider how different it feels to eat dinner in a formal dining room compared to propped up in bed or perched on a picnic blanket at the beach. Even the shape and size of a table can affect the ambiance. Eating at a round table, with no one presiding at either end and individuals sitting roughly equidistant from one another, feels more egalitarian than eating at a rectangular table. Proximity or distance of the seats can also alter the dining experience. Sitting at a table that's a tight squeeze may promote more intimate conversation than one where everyone has plenty of legroom.

In the film *Citizen Kane,* Orson Welles shows the deterioration of a marriage using the changing size of a dining room table to mirror the increasing emotional distance of a couple. The first scene shows a young couple sitting next to each other at a small table, engaged in romantic banter. In each successive scene, the tabletop becomes more crowded and the couple is seated farther apart. In the ninth and final scene, they are sitting at opposite ends of a long table, reading rival newspapers—the collapse of their marriage is reflected in the spatial features of the table. Our sense of emotional closeness can be keenly felt by the physical space between us at the table. Often, a smaller table feels more conducive to easy conversation.

When I talk with families about their dinners, most tell me the same thing: Each family member sits in the same chair night after night. No one can quite remember how these decisions were made. But in most families, it is considered a subversive act to claim a seat that isn't customarily yours. In my husband's family, the girls sat on one side of the table, nearer the stove, so that they could spring up to help with food, while the boys sat on the far side. As with most rectangular tables, his parents sat at either end, connoting higher status as heads of the table.

What would happen if you asked family members to choose a seat that wasn't their customary one? What if you sit very close or with more than usual distance between seats? What if you dispense with chairs altogether, and try spreading a blanket on the floor or in a different room or outside? What about turning off the lights and lighting candles?

At The Family Dinner Project community dinners, we often kick things off with kids making placemats for themselves and their parents, or by creating centerpieces out of a motley array of random objects—feathers, pipe cleaners, rocks, and flowers. This purposeful setting of the table seems to pave the way for a new experience at the community dinner.

You can do this at home with sheets of computer or easel paper. If you are feeling more ambitious, you can cut pieces of fabric (hemming them so they don't fray) and use fabric pens. Have everyone draw pictures of the family, or self-portraits, or portraits of someone else at the table (then you have to find the seat that has your picture). Or draw maps of your neighborhood, or pictures of something you really love to do. If there are creations you want to keep, you can get them laminated and reuse them for special occasions, or even for a tired Wednesday night.

PLAY WITH MUSIC

Given that most teenagers will listen to about 6,000 hours of music between the ages of twelve and eighteen,[5] there are a lot of stories and language that they will be privy to through listening to songs. I think that parents who want access to their kids' inner lives may learn a lot by listening to their children's music. A CD or playlist of your child's current favorite music, played at dinner, can be a great way to do this, and you have your teen right there to help interpret what you're listening to.

Another idea is to create a compilation of songs about food that can make for inspiring music during cooking and cleanup time. You might start with some classics such as "Food, Glorious Food" and Cab Calloway's "Everyone Eats When They Come to My House." I'd also include The Band's "Up on Cripple Creek," which has the memorable line, "dip a donut in my tea," as well as Van Morrison's "Tupelo Honey" and Dr. John's "Jambalaya."

Lynn Barendsen, the executive director of The Family Dinner Project, shared a music game she plays with her husband and two sons. One person throws out a word, like "car," and then everyone tries to come up with a song that has the word in the lyrics or the title: Bruce Springsteen's song, "Fire" with the line, "I'm driving in my car," and Tracy Chapman's "Fast Car" are two examples. Then the family tries to sing a bit of the song.

PLAY FOOD GAMES

My friend Bev is a member of a large Asian-American family in the Boston area. Every summer, for the past thirty years, she and her four siblings have rented a house together for a long "sibling weekend" so that they wouldn't lose touch with one another as they became busy with careers and families and were spread out across the country. As the decades have unspooled, children and grandparents have been added to the mix. This summer visit is sacrosanct, and everyone manages to show up, which isn't possible for the big holidays when in-laws compete for family time.

When I asked Bev what they like to do together, she told me that everyone likes to eat and play games. One sister, Patty, is the major games leader, organizing everything from Olympics to word games, and everyone pitches in with the cooking.

One recent summer, in Deering, New Hampshire, when their ranks had swelled to nineteen, cooking and gaming converged for a rousing version of the popular competitive TV cooking show *Iron Chef.* Bev and another sister were team captains, choosing their teams as though it were a game of pick-up basketball. (For other games, the family divides itself into first-borns and later-borns, but according to Bev, who is the second of five, the later-borns almost always win because they are better at collaborating with one another).

For the family-wide game of Iron Chef, Patty played the role of judge, also picking three ingredients that had to be incorporated into the meal:

salmon, potatoes, and peaches. Everyone participated throughout the afternoon, peeling potatoes and peaches, and negotiating about what dishes they should create. Bev recalls that her team found pastel-colored glasses and filled them with peach daiquiris. Then there was a potato soup and baked salmon (decorated with fins and gills made out of roasted potatoes). For dessert they wanted to make Nora Ephron's "Best Peach Pie," from *Heartburn,* but thought it was out of reach since they'd left the book at home. One of the kids easily found it online.

The other team made salmon sashimi (garnished with lemons and herbs from the garden) as an appetizer, salmon with peach salsa as the main dish, and grilled peaches with balsamic vinegar and crème fraiche. When it came to judging the two meals, Patty decided that it was best not to declare a winner but to give out commendations, for best drink, presentation, originality, and so on. Bev agreed that this was a wise move. "We're a very competitive family," she said.

PLAY WITH SCIENCE, PART 1

Preschoolers to age eight

Young children love to make concoctions from leftover food, soap bubbles, seltzer water, and spoonfuls of sugar, salt, and other baking items. The unexpected chemical reactions that ensue create bubbling and fizzing, strange aromas, and weird colors—all reactions that need to be closely supervised. (After all, you don't want your kids to eat or drink these brews.) My kids made these by the hour at the kitchen sink and in our driveway when they got too messy for the kitchen. Joe even bottled them and set up a stand on our street, hawking them as magical elixirs. A kindly neighbor bought one, which only egged Joe on. If you want to guide your children toward more purposeful chemistry projects, here are a few that are fun:

PLAY DOUGH

2 cups flour
1 cup salt

2 cups water
4 teaspoons cream of tartar
2 tablespoons vegetable oil
Food coloring

Mix all of the ingredients together in a bowl, except for the food coloring. Plunk the mixture into a pot, and stir over very low heat until a ball forms. When you remove it from the heat, you can separate the dough into smaller balls, and add different drops of food coloring to each ball. While there is nothing toxic about this dough, it will induce great thirst from its high salt content. Nibbling, while tempting, should probably be kept to a minimum.

SOAP

A few bars of glycerin soap (available online or at a crafts store)
Essential oil (available online or at a bath and body shop). Use any fragrance you like—lavender and mint work nicely.
Food coloring or natural color, such as juice or cinnamon
Molds: paper cups, yogurt cups, or plastic containers
Whimsical objects (optional): a leaf, a flower, and a small plastic trinket

Melt the soaps in the top of a double boiler over boiling water. (I used a beat-up pot, bought at a yard sale.) Add the essential oil. Next add a few drops of color. Pour the mixture into a mold. For extra zip, you can add a whimsical object, which will reveal itself when the soap melts. Once the soap hardens, tear the paper or cut the plastic off the soap. These make very nice holiday gifts.

SUGAR WATER FOR BRIGHTER CHALK

½ cup water
2 tablespoons sugar

Mix together the ingredients in a small bowl. Dip chalk into the mixture. You'll find that your chalk drawings are brighter and less smudgy when you go to make hopscotch courts and pictures on the sidewalk.

PLAY WITH SCIENCE, PART 2

School-age kids and teenagers

One hot July afternoon, I descended into the basement of an engineering building on the Harvard campus to visit a food and science camp for kids ages nine to twelve. Geoff Lukas, the chef de cuisine at one of my favorite restaurants, Sofra, had invited me to attend his one-hour class within this weeklong camp. Sofra—a friendly restaurant with imaginative dishes from all across the Mediterranean—is situated across the street from the Mount Auburn Cemetery in Watertown, Massachusetts. I had already learned a lot from Geoff when he taught a class there about cooking with flowers. He is also a master of pickling.

At the Harvard Food and Science Camp, Geoff presented each child with an array of pickled foods:

- Amba (a fermented green mango with salt, cumin, coriander, garlic, and onion)
- A pickled green strawberry (a ripe red strawberry will produce too much fizzing from the high sugar content)
- Garlic that had been pickled for more than a year (turned green to blue to brown)
- An acid pickle (white wine vinegar with spices, poured over cucumber until cooked all the way through)
- A fermented pickle (a salt solution that doesn't involve cooking and results in a mellower flavor than the acid pickle)
- Sauerkraut (shredded cabbage with salt that draws out the water)

While the kids tasted this pickled bounty (with many noses wrinkled in disgust), Geoff explained the scientific processes at work, which involve microbes eating sugar to produce lactic acid. I feared that the sour taste of the pickles combined with the technicality of the teaching might fall flat on this group of about twenty-five kids. Boy, was I wrong.

One hand shot up as soon as Geoff stopped cooking. Peter, a ten-year-old boy from Cambridge, with a Milky Way constellation of freckles across the bridge of his nose, asked how Geoff's pickles compared to bread-and-butter pickles. (Apparently bread-and-butter pickles are a type of acid pickle with a lot of turmeric and sugar). Soon, hands were popping up across the room. Is there a time limit for pickling? Would nine years be too long? What is the weirdest thing you've ever pickled? Can you pickle bread, water, ice cream, or something with a peel? (Yes, to this last list of items.)

Later, I chatted more with Peter, who has been making pickles for years. He's already tried pickling apples and peaches and couldn't wait to pickle avocados, which he predicted would taste like salty ice cream. He told me that he keeps a doodle pad, where he records all of his cooking experiments.

"I like to mess things up with baking," he said. "If I'm making a raspberry cake, I'll make everything raspberry—the cake, the chocolate filling and the topping—and see how that tastes." It seemed that in the course of Peter's food play, he was also a budding scientist. By changing ingredients, he was able to see what difference those variations made to a recipe. Maybe he was more of an artist than a methodical scientist who changes one element at a time in a recipe to see what longer cooking time, more butter, vanilla instead of chocolate, will do to a cake recipe. But still, the process of trial and error, observation and testing, and then recording the results is at the heart of the scientific process. By playing with their food, Peter and the other kids in the camp were getting training as young scientists.

Here are two pickling recipes from Chef Geoff Lukas:

PICKLED SUNGOLD TOMATOES (ORANGE CHERRY TOMATOES)

1 pint Sungold tomatoes
2 (1-inch) sprigs rosemary

½ cup honey (preferably a lighter variety, like a spring blossom)

½ cup champagne vinegar

½ cup water

1 teaspoon salt

Wash the tomatoes and remove any remaining stems. Lay them out on a cloth or paper towel to prevent residual water from diluting the liquid. Prick each tomato with a needle or push pin (this will keep the tomatoes from bursting in the liquid). Place the tomatoes and the rosemary in a heat-proof container. Combine the remaining ingredients in a small pot and bring to a full boil, stirring well. Allow the liquid to cool 5 minutes and pour over the tomatoes. They should sit at least overnight, but the flavors will deepen and mellow over time. Refrigerated, they will keep at least one month.

SOUR CUCUMBERS (BASIC BRINING METHOD)

Spices (1 tablespoon peppercorns, 1 tablespoon mustard seed,
    ½ tablespoon allspice, ½ tablespoon coriander)

¼ cup torn sprigs dill

5 tablespoons salt (preferably an unrefined salt like gray salt or
    Maldon salt)

2 quarts water

3 pounds cucumbers, whole and unpeeled

1 bulb garlic (cut at the bottom to expose the cloves)

Toast the spices until they are aromatic. Combine the spices, dill, salt, and water in a bowl, stirring vigorously to combine. The brine will take some extra whisking to ensure that the larger grains of salt are dissolved.

Wash the cucumbers and pat dry. Place the cucumbers and the garlic in a fermentation vessel (described below). Pour the brine over the vegetables.

Ideally, the vegetables will be stored at 65°F to 75°F. Fermentation should start within two to three days. The vegetables will be half-sour in about a week and fully fermented in about two weeks. Properly stored, they will keep almost indefinitely, and the flavors will develop with time. If temperature control is not possible, allow the fermentation to start and, once bubbling is seen, move the cucumbers to the refrigerator and allow to sit at least two weeks.

Key points to know about fermenting

Airtight ceramic, nonreactive metal, or food-grade plastic are the ideal vessels for fermentation. The produce should be fully submerged in brine, held down with either a weight or a screen. Airtight is important because air is the enemy and will cause mold growth and other defects.

The proportion of produce to water to salt is very important. The brine, in the previous recipe, is about 5 percent salt (by weight of the water). Cucumbers are about 95 percent water (whereas carrots, for example, are about 70 percent). This dictates how much the produce itself will dilute the solution through osmosis. The salt can be varied slightly to taste, but 3 percent is a pretty strict minimum, particularly in hotter storage conditions. When varying the recipe, either for personal preference or for other produce, care must be taken to observe safe minimums.

FISH TACOS (FOR 4)

Created by my son Joe, this is a delicious use of pickles in a dish. He ate a version of these from a food truck on the Lower East Side in Manhattan. Re-creating a dish at home that you've tasted at a restaurant (or food truck) is another kind of food play.

2 tablespoons white or champagne wine vinegar
1 tablespoon sugar
½ teaspoon salt
½ red onion, thinly sliced
1 pint cherry tomatoes
½ red onion, finely diced
Juice of 2 limes

Salt and pepper

1 avocado

¼ cup mayonnaise

1 teaspoon lime juice

1 cup all-purpose flour

Cayenne pepper to taste

¼ cup canola oil

1 pound cod fillets or other firm white fish

1 (8-count) small package soft corn tortillas

Mix the vinegar, sugar, and salt in a small bowl. Pour the mixture over the sliced red onions and let sit for at least one hour. This creates a very quick pickling process.

Halve the cherry tomatoes and combine them in a bowl with the finely diced red onions, the juice of two limes, salt, and pepper. (If you're feeling adventurous, add a small chopped jalapeño pepper, with seeds and ribs removed.)

Scoop out the avocado and mash it with a fork in a small bowl. Add the mayonnaise to the avocado, and mix until creamy. Season with 1 teaspoon lime juice and salt and pepper to taste.

Combine the flour, salt and pepper, and cayenne pepper in a shallow baking dish or high-rimmed plate. Slice the cod into 3-inch-long chunks. Dredge the fish in the flour mixture. Be sure to remove any clumps of flour that adhere to the fish, since these will just burn in the pan.

Heat the canola oil in a frying pan over high heat. (Don't be afraid of cranking up your stove to the highest flame and watching the oil smoke.) Place the cod into the pan, making sure not to overcrowd it, which will bring down the temperature in the pan. Fry for 2 minutes on each side. Any more will dry out the fish and make it rubbery.

Just before serving, heat the tortillas in a dry saucepan over low heat.

Now it's time to assemble the tacos. Spread the avocado cream in a thin layer on each tortilla shell. You'll need two tacos per person. Place a piece of cod on the avocado spread. Top the fish with the cherry tomato salsa and pickled onions.

Making food is a form of play that can engage the whole family and it may be the only experience we still have at home that involves touching, smelling, and manipulating real objects. As our worlds have become more virtual, the creative act of making food takes on special meaning. If we still built chairs, made quilts, chopped down trees, and hauled water from the well, then perhaps cooking wouldn't be quite so meaningful. But cooking remains that rare activity that still involves our senses and our hands, and it is something that we still can do together.

Its colors and textures create opportunities for artistic expression. Its chemical properties permit scientific experimentation and dramatic trans-formations. The language around food is ripe with puns and multiple meanings. The context of eating is also available to have fun with as you play with seating and music.

I'm sure that my examples of play represent only a small sampling of the possibilities that exist. I haven't even touched the potential fun of baking bread, churning ice cream, or making pasta. Whether you come to food with a scientific sensibility or an artistic flair, I hope that playing with your food will lead to many extra hours of fun with your fellow cooks.

6

Table Talk That Goes Beyond "How Was Your Day?"

I n most families, the bread and butter of dinnertime talk centers around the question, "How was your day?" In some families, this simple question opens the floodgates: Kids will talk about recess, or about a rebuke someone endured from a teacher, or about an intriguing moral dilemma that arose in class. But some kids will only respond with a one-word answer: "Okay." In other families, one member grabs all the airtime and rattles off a string of anecdotes about what happened during the day; meanwhile, everyone else will be tapping toes, impatient to get a word in edgewise.

In this chapter, I give some suggestions about how to overcome these and other table talk challenges so that you can increase your family members' desire to talk and also to listen to each other.

Even if you're lucky enough to have family members who need little prompting to gush about their days, it can be interesting and fun to raise some other topics for discussion. A steady diet of "how was your day" questions can feel like eating the same meal night after night. So, like switching up the menu, it's good to add some variety and surprise. Games can be used to extend the time families spend with each other and infuse table talk with a dollop of playfulness. Dinnertime is also an opportunity to talk about things that matter—items in the news or abstract issues that encourage family members to think about what they would do in a similar situation.

The dinner table is also the primary place that families tell stories about parents and previous generations, stories that transmit the idea that we are all part of something bigger than ourselves. (Because this topic is so important, I'm giving it its own chapter: Chapter 7.)

ENCOURAGING TALKING AND LISTENING

Sometimes getting your kids to participate in dinner conversation feels like a lost cause, but you'll be surprised at how easy it becomes when you use some simple, but effective techniques.

Asking questions that elicit more than a one-word answer

Kids have many good reasons for answering their parents' questions with one word. It could be that they've been answering questions all day and now want a break, or they're so tired and hungry that one word is all they can muster, or they've got a lot on their minds and the question you've asked isn't interesting enough to change their focus. They could also be upset about something and don't want to share it, or they just plain don't feel like talking but wouldn't mind listening to *you* talk.

Of course, it's impossible to know what's going on if your child won't tell you, and that's the catch-22. Here are a few ideas that have worked with my children over the years, as well as with child patients of mine who are very prone to clamming up in a therapist's office. I can't guarantee that these ideas are foolproof or that each idea will work for every child every time. You know your child well enough to predict which, if any, of these approaches might help get the conversation flowing.

- Keep a "map" in your head of what you know transpired in your child's day, and ask questions that demonstrate that you have been paying attention. In other words, ask a question that shows that the details of your child's life matter enough for you to have remembered them. For example, "I know that today was your first art class. What was it like?" or "Did you have a chance to play 'monkey in the middle' again at recess like you did yesterday? Whom did you play with today?" (This notion of keeping an updated map is a good idea with fellow adults as well. I know I find it maddening if my husband forgets to ask me about a big presentation and starts a conversation with a clueless, "How was your day, hon?")

- As your day rolls along, try collecting small stories that might interest or amuse your children, such as something mischievous the dog did during the day or a funny exchange with a coworker. Later, when you reunite with your child, you might start with a story of your own. Often, this kind of modeling helps gets the ball rolling, and it shows your child that you are offering something before asking for something.

- Ask questions that require only one-word answers but not necessarily just yes or no. For example, "What did you like better today, math or reading?" "Who was most fun to play with today? And then who?" Sometimes, kids realize that they are offering information anyway and decide to fill in more of the details.

- In graduate school I was taught a saying about how to make certain behaviors, like one-word answers, less attractive to patients. The saying is "Spit in the soup." That means, by predicting that your child is going to do the very thing that you wish she wouldn't, you lessen the appeal of her likely behavior—so it's like soup that's been spoiled by spitting in it. For example, you might say "Sally, I want to ask you about your day, and I know that you're only going to want to give me a one-word answer, but that's okay; that's all I really expect right now."

- Take a break from asking questions and instead wonder out loud about parts of your child's day without asking anything. "At noon today I was thinking about you because I knew you were trying out for the school play, and I was hoping that all the rehearsing you did last night made you feel confident." Then just be quiet, and see if your child adds on to what you've started.

And, then there's the more direct approach. You can always ask your children to help you be better at having a conversation about their day. "I'm so excited to see you, and so interested in what you've been doing, what you're learning, and who you've played with, but often you don't seem to want to talk. Is there anything that makes it easier or harder for you to share some of your day with me?"

Your child might answer, "Yes, don't ask me so many questions!" Then you can wonder aloud what she might not like about your questions. If you figure it out, you might be on your way to changing the conversation.

DEEPENING THE CONVERSATION

As my kids would certainly tell you, I can be a real pest when it comes to asking questions. My husband, a journalist, is no better. Since we both ask questions for a living, our kids have been interrogated, quizzed, and cross-examined within an inch of their lives. In my defense, I do try to ask a broad range of questions—some to get the facts, others that wonder about feelings, and still others to try to pivot around an issue by asking a question from a different perspective.

Some questions and responses are like oxygen, keeping the flame of conversation alive; others are sure to throw cold water on it. I'm sure I've thrown more than my share of cold-water on dinnertime discussions, but I aspire to be a human bellows. Here are some ways to keep a conversation alive.

Let's consider this simple exchange—likely happening at dinner tables across the country—to compare the two different types of communication. A parent asks: What was the best thing that happened at school today?" The child responds: "Recess."

Responses that shut down the conversation

- *Negatively judging your child's response.* "Didn't you learn anything in class today? Do you think school is all fun and games?"
- *Persuading or cajoling your child to consider a different response.* "Are you really sure that was the best thing about school today? I seem to

remember that you were going to have a parent come in today to read a story; wasn't that more fun than recess?"

- *Making the response a problem.* "Why were you so relieved to get away from class and into recess? Did something bad happen in class today?"

Questions that fan the flames of conversation

- *Asking out of pure curiosity* and conveying that you want to understand your child's point of view. "Tell me more. What did you do? Whom did you play with?"
- *Asking playful questions that introduce a different perspective.* "If I had been a bee on the swing, what would I have seen?"
- *Asking your child to compare two experiences.* "How was recess today different from recess yesterday? Was there something that made it particularly fun today?"
- *Asking questions that prompt your child to talk about his or her successes.* "Did you do something during recess that you were particularly proud of or that you want to remember to do again?"
- *Asking questions that shine light on what's missing.* If your child talks about feelings, you might ask: "What were you thinking about?" If your child talked about today, you could ask about tomorrow or yesterday.
- *Inviting others into the conversation.* "Recess makes me think of taking a break during the day. What kinds of breaks did others take during the day? What are your favorite ways to relax and recharge during the day?"

And don't forget that you won't be the only one generating questions. Children are question-asking engines. I'm sure you know this from your own experience, but to give you an idea of *just* how much kids enjoy asking questions, consider this 2007 study: A researcher analyzed more than 200 hours of recordings of four kids, between the ages of two and five, talking with their caregivers. On average, the kids asked one to three questions per minute, or about 75 per hour![1]

Sometimes it might be helpful to wonder out loud what it is you don't know. For example, "I'm not sure I really understand Snapchat. Could you tell me about it?" By embracing "not knowing," you may come up with some of the best fan-flaming questions.

MANAGING CONFLICT

Once the talk starts flowing, conflict and fighting could erupt. Some families enjoy having animated discussions at the dinner table, airing out different political views or replaying an umpire's call at last night's ballgame. Jack, a middle-aged man, and one of three sons, reflected on his childhood dinners: "Fighting with Dad about the Vietnam War was a sport that we all looked forward to. We sharpened our wits at the table. My father made each of us feel that we were worthy opponents, and I liked that."

Speaking in a forthright way about differing opinions can make family members feel that each person's individuality is valued and that the table is a safe place to send up a challenge. But if you want to tone down the conflict at the table to make room for other types of conversations, here are some tips:

- *Agree to keep off the table topics that usually result in a fight.* It may be easier to discuss such issues as grades, curfew, and behavior problems *after* dinner—on a full stomach and once you've had a chance to reconnect.
- *Go easy on teaching manners at the table.* You have years to remedy behaviors like kids eating with their hands and blowing bubbles in their milk. But it's hard for kids to relax when they're constantly being corrected. And it's not so easy for parents to enjoy dinnertime if they have to be constantly vigilant about their children's manners. So focus on one priority at a time, and don't let the enforcement of minding manners take over the dinner. You can, though, focus on the manners that help build respectful speaking and listening, like not speaking with your mouth full, or not talking over anyone. Those are manners that we can all try to improve, so kids won't feel so singled out.

- *Set some guidelines for conversation, if necessary, such as "Only one person can speak at a time" or "We're not going to interrupt each other."* One large, talkative family has the rule that family members can talk only if they are holding a shell. When they are done speaking, the shell is passed to the next speaker.

- *Complaining about the food is one of the greatest sources of conflict at the table.* Nothing sours my mood more quickly than cooking a dinner that my sons don't like. When they were young I circumvented this source of conflict by preparing a list of meals that everyone agreed to eat without bellyaching. From time to time I would update the list. Then I would know that they had signed off on any meal I was taking the time to prepare.

- *Using technology at the table is another growing source of family tension.* A 2012 survey found that there are two sets of standards at the dinner table.[2] Parents use technology at the table at twice the rate that their children are allowed. In other words, what's good for the goose isn't so good for the gosling. Perhaps a starting point would be for parents and kids to agree on the rules. The rules might well be a no-technology policy at the table, so that face-to-face conversation is consistently valued. Other families might agree to use technology lightly but only to share content with fellow diners, not to text with absent parties.

- *Managing "that's not fair" complaints.* Where there are siblings there are almost always complaints about fairness. My sons, who are two and a half years apart, could be best friends one minute and outraged with each other the next, at a perceived inequity. When complaints, of "he got more" rang out, I would try to remind them that fairness is about getting what you need rather than getting the same amount as your brother. As my husband used to say over and over, "It's not equal, but it's fair."

PLAYING GAMES

Playing games at the table can bring variety to the conversation and can also be an effective way to extend your dinner hour. I favor playing games that don't require any boards, dice, or screens because those items can add complications, like spilling milk on an iPad or losing a game piece in a bowl of soup.

For children under age eight

There are many word games that are fun to play at the table, and can then lead to interesting conversations even after the game is over.

ROSE AND THORN　　This is a game that really works for all ages, and it is one of our go-to games at The Family Dinner Project community dinners because it's so user-friendly. (It's also a game that, according to numerous media sources, the Obama family plays at their family dinners.) Each family member describes something positive (the rose of the day) and something negative or difficult (the thorn). I like the way this game puts everyone on the same level and gives a structured way to talk about what can feel amorphous. There are countless variations on this question if your family gets bored with this version. You can ask for the silliest and most serious thing that happened, the most surprising thing that happened, or what made you feel happy, impatient, grateful, annoyed, or some other attitude that might engage the members of your family.

GUESS THAT EMOTION　　This is a game that's fun for younger kids. It has the added bonus of helping kids identify feelings, which is a building block in developing the capacity for empathy.

As a family, you might first brainstorm several examples of feelings—like sad, angry, happy, surprised, worried, excited—and agree that the game will be based on this list. (This will cut down on family members wanting to use more obscure and hard-to-enact states, such as agitated or stunned). Have one person volunteer to leave the table for a minute. Once she leaves, the rest of the family decides on an emotion. When she returns, the rest of the family talks and eats with that feeling in mind but without naming the emotion. The family member who is in the dark has to guess what emotion is being enacted.

For example, if the emotion is "worried" someone might say, "I think you'll bite my head off if I get up to get another helping of soup," and a child might say, "I have so much homework to do tonight, I'm never going to get to sleep." Or if the emotion is "happy," a parent might say, "That soup was so delicious, I can't wait to have some more," and another family member might declare, "I am really enjoying the conversation we're having tonight." Each family member can take a turn leaving the room and guessing the emotion. You can play this game with older children as well and kick up the difficulty by allowing only body language or facial expression to convey the emotion.

TWO TRUTHS AND A TALL TALE   This game is another one that we play at The Family Dinner Project community dinners, like the one we held in Lynn, Massachusetts, with six families, including children who ranged from toddlers to teens. I think it is intriguing to adults as well as kids.

Each person comes up with two factual statements about himself or his experiences and one that is a fiction. The three statements are presented to the family, and everyone has to guess which item has been made up. Of course, trying to disguise a false item is particularly challenging for family members who know each other very well, but keep in mind that the game can also be used to start a conversation about what happened during the day. For example: "For lunch I ate a piece of chocolate cake and a yogurt; I walked up nine flights to my office because the elevator was broken; and I learned something new today about yoga."

MINDFULNESS GAME   Ask all your diners to close their eyes and remain silent for about a minute while you ask them to focus on what they hear and what they smell. Children generally have more acute senses of hearing and smell than adults do, so don't be surprised if the kids identify things that don't register for the adults. For added fun, encourage everyone to imitate the sounds they hear or try to describe the smells. This game is enriched by playing it outside while picnicking so you're privy to sounds other than the ticking of a clock or the whirring of a refrigerator motor.

GUESS THE TITLE   This is a game I adapted from Jay Allison's 60-second Shortlist spots on WCAI, the public radio station on Cape Cod and the Islands. A short list is made "from your experience or research or daily life."

(In the radio version, the list is read out loud and then, after a pause, the listener hears what the list was all about.) If I were to be on the radio I might offer the following: sleeping late, sand in my sheets, no TV, outdoor shower, riding the waves, losing sunglasses, ice cream cones dipped in chocolate, no to-do lists. Then there would be a pause so the listener could conjure up the title of my list: "A beach vacation."

For kids of all ages, this more pedestrian version of shortlists works well: Each person lists a bunch of items, tangible or not, and then the rest of the family has to guess what the intended title of the list might be. For example, an adult might list: loose change, a car key, tissues, lipstick, and a flashlight. The title turns out to be "contents of my pocketbook." A child might compose a list of "foods I hate" or "countries I want to visit in my lifetime."

When we've played this game at The Family Dinner Project community dinners, we've adapted it for preschool children. A parent might whisper a category to them—say, things in your bed or favorite things to do in the summer—and have them list the items out loud so that the others can guess the title.

WOULD YOU RATHER   Here's a game I learned from The Family Dinner Project team. Each family member takes a turn asking "Would you rather . . ." questions. Of course you can make up your own, but to get you started, here are a few from our team. *Would you rather . . .*

   ___ be able to fly or be invisible?
   ___ speak every language in the world or play every instrument?
   ___ live in the future or the past?
   ___ live without a phone or without a TV?
   ___ lose your sense of taste or your sense of smell?
   ___ go to the beach in the summer or skiing in the winter?
   ___ meet the president of the United States or your favorite movie star?
   ___ live in the city or the country?
   ___ have to eat a bowl of crickets or a bowl of worms?
   ___ always have the same song stuck in your head or always have the
        same dream at night?

___ always have to enter the room backward or always have to somersault out?

For children eight and older

Kids who are old enough to recognize more of the foods you serve and whose verbal skills are better developed than their younger peers may enjoy the following games.

FRUIT AND VEGETABLE GAME I can play the fruit and vegetable game by the hour (and have). One family member (the "leader"of a round) thinks of a person known by everyone else at the table. Then others around the table ask the leader metaphorical questions to try guess this person. For example, "If this person were a vegetable, what vegetable would he or she be?" or "If he or she were a fruit, or a dessert, which would he or she be?" You can branch out to nonfood categories, such as "What color, animal, or type of weather would this person be?" The idea is to stick to figurative rather than literal thinking. In other words, the leader will answer in terms of how the individual's personality might be manifested in another form rather than answering in terms of the person's actual favorite vegetable to eat or color that they like to wear. Once the leader shares at least a few category examples, everyone else tries to guess the person who is being described metaphorically. The player who guesses correctly gets to think up the next person.

In therapy, I've often played this with siblings and had them come up with descriptors for their parents. It's especially interesting to them, and to me, when the images are very similar (for example, "My mother is like an orange or a peach") and when the images clash (as in "My mother is like a lemon." "No, she's more like a watermelon!") These similarities or differences can springboard a discussion about each one's perceptions of a person who, although known by all, is perhaps experienced in different ways.

HIGGLETY-PIGGLETY One person thinks of two rhyming words, such as "crazy daisy," but doesn't tell the group what he is thinking. Instead, he gives a synonym, such as "insane flower." He also lets everyone know how many syllables are in the words they're guessing by using the phrase "higglety-pigglety" (three-syllable words), or "higgy-piggy" (two-syllable words), or "hig-pig" (one-syllable words). "Crazy daisy" is a higgy-piggy, whereas "history mystery" is a "higglety-pigglety." (Naturally, for the purpose of this game, chosen words should contain no more than three syllables.) Everyone guesses, and whoever gets it first gets to think of the next one.

HOW WELL DO YOU KNOW ME?   Another game I've played with much hilarity with young teen boys (not the easiest group to involve in a table game) and with three generations of my family is the "How well do you know me?" game. You pass out slips of blank paper to each person at the table and ask them to answer three questions. The leader comes up with the questions, which are infinite in possibility, and preferably a bit whimsical. Some examples are: "If your house was burning, what is one item you would grab?," "If you could have dinner with a celebrity, who would that be?," and "If you could be a character in a book, what character would you be?"

Once each participant has written down three responses, the leader of the game collects all the slips of paper. She then reads aloud each person's response to the first question while everyone tries to guess which answer corresponds with which person. As an example, with five players, let's say you're reading all the answers to the prompt "What tattoo would you put on your neck?" The answers are: a bluebird, a heart, my birth date, a skull, and a mathematical equation. After each person guesses which response goes with which player, a correct guess scores a point. But, honestly, the game is entertaining enough that you don't even need to keep score—unless you're playing this with young teen boys and then maybe you do!

FOOD WORD GAME   When my kids were in elementary school, one son was given the assignment to come up with as many words as he could that related to birds. I hope it wasn't cheating when we all spent hours that night at the dinner table free-associating to bird words and bird-related words. We came up with hundreds. My husband is a lifelong birder, so he's as obsessed with winged creatures as I am with food.

It got me thinking: What if we played the same game with food words? How many words or expressions can you come up with that contain the word salt? (For starters—salt in the wound, salty dog, salt-and-pepper beard.) Or bread? (Bread and butter, man cannot live by bread alone.) Or fish? (Neither fish nor fowl, fishing for compliments, fish or cut bait.) You can go around the table with each person coming up with a word or phrase until you run out of options. The last person able to come up with a word scores a point.

MUSIC LYRIC GAMES   One family who had turned to The Family Dinner Project for help because their three teenagers were eating fast-food dinners in their bedrooms ended up teaching us a table game they made up. This game spontaneously emerged once the family started eating together (and enjoying healthy food). One parent would bring up an item from the news, and the kids would create rap lyrics that connected to the news item; the parents would come up with an old pop song lyric that also applied.

Another game is Name That Tune. Hum a few bars of a popular tune and see who can guess the tune first. You can use ad jingles, holiday songs, popular songs from the radio, family favorites sung on car rides, or any other song that everyone will know.

CONVERSATION STARTERS IN A JAR   This game is good for all ages. Cut up dozens of little strips of paper. On each one, write a "conversation starter." There are tons of examples offered on The Family Dinner Project website (thefamilydinnerproject.org), but here is a sampling:

"What are two things you feel grateful for today?"
"Who is your best friend?"
"If you are feeling sick or sad, what can someone do to care for you?"
"What is your favorite story about our family?"
"What is your favorite character in a book or movie? Why?"
"Do you know how your name was chosen?"
"If you had three wishes, what would they be?"
"What is your favorite thing to do outside?"

"Do you prefer to speak or to listen?"

"What is your best personality trait?"

"Where do you feel most relaxed?"

"If you could be one age for the rest of your life, what age would it be? Why?"

Then stuff these slips of paper into a jar or tissue box. When conversation lags, suggest that someone pull out a slip and answer the question. Other family members can answer the same question or pull out another one.

TALKING ABOUT THINGS THAT MATTER

How is talk supported at your table? If the conversation allows for free expression of feeling, tolerates differences of opinion, and enables everyone to feel listened to, then it *is* conversation that matters. Anything more is gravy. But since gravy enhances the flavor, let's talk about that. The gravy is talk about what's important to you as a family, and as individuals. It's also conversation about moral dilemmas that test how you want to live your lives.[3] With my children, some of the best conversations we've had were prompted by ethical dilemmas that my husband or I faced in the course of an ordinary day. I remember my husband telling our sons, then early adolescents, that he had caught a student cheating on a test. He knew that by turning him in the student would likely lose his scholarship and have to drop out. What should he do? (He ended up giving him an F on the test and a very stern lecture that was meant to scare some sense into the young man.)

Another approach taken by Amy Chua, Yale law professor and author of *Battle Hymn of the Tiger Mother,* is to pose hypothetical moral challenges to her children: "If one of us committed a crime, would you turn us in?"[4] Historical events that your kids are studying can also be good fodder for conversation. "What do you think we could have done as a family if we wanted to protect a Jewish friend during Hitler's rise to power?" Obviously, neither of these conversational prompts makes for light chitchat, nor would they be suitable for children who are younger than about twelve.

If you're looking for a continual source of interesting conversation, look no further than daily media content. For example, elections can prompt discussions about how democracy works and what it means when people have to wait for hours to vote. Scandals can provide fodder for talk about truth telling. News about an abusive coach can prompt conversation about what inspires players to play better and what behavior is off-limits.

On The Family Dinner Project's website, the "Conversation of the Week" offers excellent examples of items in the news that can provide the springboard for lively conversations at the table.

If you want to provoke conversations about ethics, you can tie those to events on the calendar. For example, on Thanksgiving talk about what kind of giving family you are or want to be, or to what groups your ancestors have given money or time. If you were to volunteer as a family, what kind of organization would you choose to help out with—one that provides medical care, food, scholarships, clothing, or human rights? Do you want to give time or money to a small or a large organization? One that is local, national, or international? One that benefits children, families, or animals?

Memorial Day, the last Monday of May, is the holiday commemorating the men and women who have died while serving in the U.S. armed forces. As well as marking the unofficial start of summer, the occasion can also be an opportunity to talk about what causes or circumstances warrant a call to war. It can prompt questions about what kind of resistance responses are warranted if our country participates in a war that you think is morally questionable.

Labor Day, another Monday holiday, celebrates the rights of American workers. It could be the chance to ask about what rights you think workers should have and which ones are most important to you.

In my roundup of different sources of dinner conversation—from news items to questions about what happened at school, from word games to guessing games, from questions about holidays to ones about historical events—I've left the most obvious conversation prompt for last. The food! Conversation about the food comprises an estimated 20 to 30 percent of mealtime talk.[5] For example, "Please pass the pepper" or "This pasta is overcooked." It is not always obvious how to stretch these kinds of remarks into full-fledged conversations. But you can ask your kids to imagine what could improve the taste of the dinner, or ask them to brainstorm other meals that could use the same ingredients. You can also ask them to think of all the people who were involved in getting a particular food to this dinner, starting with the farmer and progressing to the truck driver, the shelf stocker at the grocery store, the checkout person, and Dad, who cooked the potatoes. And, as a last conversation topic, there's always "What shall we have for dinner tomorrow night?"

7

Telling Stories to Promote Empathy, Self-Esteem, Resilience, and Enjoyment

I f good food brings us to the table, it's often stories that make us linger long after the last piece of pie is gone. Stories are created in many flavors: fairy tales, ghost stories, thrillers, whodunits, tales of heroism, and happily-ever-after romances. But the stories told around real-life dinner tables tend to be of two distinct and special varieties: stories that family members tell about recent events that happened at school or at work and family stories about things that happened sometime in the past, often many decades earlier.

It's intriguing to think about the fact that, in a given family, thousands of stories are told, yet only a small subset of those get retold, and an even smaller subset of those gets passed to the next generation. Let's consider a family of four and their story-generating capability: If each member tells one story a night for eighteen years, they will have come up with more than 25,000 stories. Yet only a fraction of those will enter the family's portfolio of favorite tales. Those that are told over and over again often convey important beliefs that a family holds dear—for example, the belief that we make our own luck or the importance of never giving up.

Family stories that get told and retold are keepsakes, in many ways more precious than a diamond pin or antique table. While I can't remember the plots of books I read last week, I could tell you dozens of stories about family members going back many generations. Of course none of these stories would be nearly as interesting as your own stories. And the reason you'll prefer your stories to mine is the same reason I can remember so many tales from my own family: They're essential to who we are.

No matter how old we are, telling stories, often with the input of others, is the primary way we make sense of the world. In fact, our brains are wired to understand one another through stories. Medical students learn about illnesses by reading case histories. Legal arguments are more convincing when they're constructed as narratives. And when it comes to children, the research says that kids who know stories about their family history have higher self-esteem and well-being.[1] Families used to spin yarns around the fire, swap tales over needlepoint, and even write letters that included stories about themselves and their neighbors. But in twenty-first-century America, the primary place where families get to share stories is the dinner table.

Family stories about the past are typically not the meat and potatoes of dinner. In one study of middle-class, two-parent families with children between the ages of nine and twelve, only 12 percent of stories told at dinner were about family history. A vast majority of stories were about the day's events.[2] But just because families don't spend a lot of time telling stories about family members, don't imagine it means that these occasional stories don't have a big impact.

Storytelling is a vital practice for people of all ages. Let's take a look at how it changes as a child grows up.

THE BENEFITS OF STORYTELLING FOR YOUNG CHILDREN

When I used to pick up my older son from preschool, he wanted to go straight to the nearby playground to swing on the monkey bars. Once he was moving fluidly from bar to bar, he'd start telling me a story about a family of raccoons. And if I listened carefully, I could hear the important nuggets of what had happened that day in school—what my son was worrying about, what he felt proud of, and what he was trying to master. In some of these stories the raccoons got into a fight and a teacher had to break it up, or a raccoon got lost and was scared he wouldn't get found, or the smallest raccoon did something very brave that surprised his parents. Maybe it was the physical release my son experienced from swinging on monkey bars that accounted for his almost always leaving the playground in a happy mood. But I think it was his storytelling.

For a young person, the very act of telling a story is powerful. For the time that he has the floor (or the monkey bars), he has captured the attention of an important person in his life. He is master of the universe! Telling stories—just like playing with Legos, dolls, or action figures—is a form of play. But instead of playing with toys, telling stories involves playing with words to make sense of the world. When children tell a story about something difficult that happened to them, they gain some mastery over the event. When they make up a story, they can try on the perspective of another person (or creature) and craft an ending that they find satisfying.

For young children, storytelling confers intellectual benefits as well as emotional ones. Telling stories around the table is linked directly to young children becoming good readers. For starters, when adults tell a story, they often include more grown-up vocabulary than you're likely to find in a children's picture book or in questions about the child's day. The parent folds in new words, knowing that the children will glean the meaning from the context of the story. Or a child may be motivated to stop the story and ask the meaning of the word, so that she can make better sense of the story being told. Preschoolers who have large vocabularies, particularly those including rare words (those not found on the 3,000 Most Common Words List), grow up to be better readers than children with more limited vocabularies.[3]

The benefits don't come just from listening to stories: Young children who know how to tell a story also have an easier time learning to read.[4] In one large study, kindergarteners who were able to tell stories grew up to be fourth- and even seventh-graders with higher reading comprehension than did those kindergarteners who lacked narrative skills.[5]

What can explain this connection between kids having early storytelling skills and later facility with reading? Perhaps they have a leg up because they develop better vocabularies through hearing and then telling stories.

Having an appetite for and then early competence in storytelling can also motivate children to dive into reading so they can learn more stories.

TEACHING CHILDREN HOW TO BECOME STORYTELLERS

By the time children are two years old, they begin to have the capacity to tell stories about themselves, particularly about a past event. And by four years old, most children understand that a good story should have a beginning, middle, and end. Preschoolers are able to report memories of events that took place more than a year earlier, but they often need adults to prompt them in recalling information about the past.[6]

In fact, parents play a key role in helping children develop their narrative skills. Imagine a parent asking a young child, "Do you remember when we went to your grandmother's house and you ate sugar candy for the first time?" This helps the child develop memory skills needed to tell a story. But that's not the only way that parents can teach their children to be raconteurs.

In a study of three-and-a-half-year-old children from economically disadvantaged families, half of the kids were assigned to a program to learn narrative skills, while others were assigned to a control group.[7] A year later, the kids in the intervention group scored higher on a vocabulary test and on a measure that assessed how much information was packed into the stories they told. Here's what the parents in the intervention group were told to do:

- Reminisce with your kids often about past experiences you have shared with them.
- Ask a lot of open-ended questions, including plenty of "when" and "where" questions rather than questions with yes and no answers.
- Encourage longer narratives by repeating what your child says or elaborating on what she says.
- Instead of deciding what story to tell, follow your child's lead in choosing what she wants to talk about.

The takeaway from this study was that children could be taught by their parents to be competent storytellers if their parents helped them elaborate and deepen their stories. And kids who could tell longer, more detailed, complex stories reaped academic benefits, such as developing bigger vocabularies.

Parents also teach narrative skills indirectly when they tell stories, particularly about events that their children also experienced. When the stories are punctuated with colorful details, suspense-filled twists of plot, and an animated presentation, children learn to recall more information of past events. Better yet, when parents include emotional words while reminiscing, children are more able to talk about feelings that they themselves have experienced.[8]

Some emotional words are more helpful than others. Research suggests that when parents point out the positive aspects of an event, even when that event is a negative one, children report higher levels of self-esteem.[9] And the best thing for kids is when parents are able to *explain* negative emotion when talking about a past event. Apparently, when kids are helped to make sense of negative emotions, such as feeling sad, angry, or scared, they develop a more positive view of themselves.

ENGAGING AND INTERESTING STORIES FOR PRESCHOOLERS

Young kids tend to be egocentric, so some of their favorite stories will star themselves or be stories about events they experienced with you. But you can use that egocentricity to guide you in your selection of family stories. For example, think back to when you were the same age as your child and tell a story from that time in your life. Perhaps you remember your first day of school or the time you got lost in a department store or got stung by a bee. Maybe you remember stories about your parents when they were small children.

Another treasure trove of possible stories involves animals, since most young children identify with small, dependent creatures. My children loved hearing their grandfather's tales of racing tortoises on the Galapagos Islands during World War II and their grandmother's story about her beloved cocker spaniel who wrote "letters" to my mother once a week, after her parents sent the dog away.

Another kind of story that is a big hit with preschoolers is a story told with lots of errors and nonsensical plot twists. Then your child can correct you with a version that makes sense. My younger son never tired of hearing me tell a story about a mother who wanted to make muffins for her family, and at each step in the recipe, she did something ridiculous, like mixing dirt and spinach in the batter, putting the muffins in a bathtub to bake, and then baking them for a week. My son would holler with indignation, and tell me not to be so silly. Then he'd correct my story so that the recipe would result in edible muffins. Better still was to top that story off by making the legitimate recipe.

MUFFINS (MAKES ABOUT A DOZEN)

1 cup old-fashioned oats

1 cup whole-wheat flour

½ cup all-purpose flour

2 teaspoons baking powder

½ teaspoon salt

¾ cup dark brown sugar

2 large eggs

¾ cup milk

¼ cup melted butter

1 teaspoon vanilla

1 cup sliced strawberries, bananas, raspberries, blueberries, chocolate chips, raisins, walnuts, or some combination (banana, chocolate chip, walnut is divine)

Mix the oats, flours, baking powder, salt, and brown sugar in a large mixing bowl. Whisk together the eggs, milk, butter, and vanilla in another, smaller bowl. Combine the dry and wet ingredients with an electric mixer. Fold in the fruit, nuts, chocolate chips, or any chosen combination.

Line a muffin tin with paper liners or grease each section with butter or oil. Fill the liners or sections with batter using an ice cream scoop. Fill about two-thirds full, so there is room at the top for the batter to rise.

Bake at 400 degrees for 15 to 20 minutes.

Young children will begin to request certain types of stories. One little girl asked her mother for "one of your funny stories" so often that her mother was afraid she was going to run out of material. Of course, most good stories can be told over and over again, and they usually morph a bit in the retelling, as the teller remembers a new detail or the listener asks a new question. Most children enjoy hearing stories about what they were like as younger versions of themselves, and most parents enjoy remembering those stories as well.

A STORYTELLING GAME

If you need a break one night from telling true stories about yourselves and your relatives, you might try this storytelling game. One person begins with a sentence and then each person at the table adds another sentence to propel the story along. The stories can feature animals, family members, teachers, neighbors, or completely made-up characters. As well as being fun, the game also enables parents to help kids learn the basic elements of any good story: a structure with a beginning, middle, interesting characters, plot twists, and suspense before the plot resolves.

STORYTELLING CAN PROMOTE EMPATHY

Children develop the capacity for empathy when they grow up feeling that someone has paid attention and really listened to them. Empathy is hard-wired into all forms of love and is, quite simply, the ability to "get" what someone else is saying and to feel that "how you feel matters to me." This capacity starts to emerge as early as toddlerhood, when children learn that they can comfort others or, for starters, their doll or stuffed animal.

Another way that empathy develops is through a child's ability to identify emotions in himself and in others. When young children have parents who talk openly about emotions, and who focus on the causes and consequences of emotion, children are better able to understand their own and other's emotions.[10]

How can empathy be fostered at the dinner table? How can kids feel well listened to and become good listeners themselves? Here are some reliable strategies:

- Make sure that everyone gets a chance to talk. Try to maintain eye contact with the person who is speaking, and don't make anyone have to compete with smartphones, TVs, or other screens while they're talking. When you have to compete, it diminishes the sense of being important enough to be listened to.
- When you tell a story, try to include the way you *felt* at different points along the way. Not only are you describing feelings, which are a foundational skill in developing empathy, but you're also telling a more interesting story. Take a look at these two stories, both true—the first, with just the facts, and the other with feelings woven in.

    Version 1: "This afternoon I was seeing a patient in my office and I heard banging overhead. At the end of the hour, I went upstairs and saw that our dog had eaten all but one of three-dozen chocolate cookies I had baked for Valentine's Day. I called the vet, who told me to give her hydrogen peroxide to make her throw up, which she did."

    Version 2: "While I was seeing a patient today, I heard banging overhead. I was terrified because I thought there was a burglar in the house. I also felt confused. Should I tell my patient that we had to stop so that I could call the police, or should I continue with the therapy and pretend that nothing was amiss? I tried to continue on, but I was so distracted and scared that I had to stop the therapy a few minutes early.

    I crept upstairs, which was pretty stupid, because what would I have done if I found an intruder? There was our dog, looking very guilty, hiding under the table, avoiding eye contact. When I saw that she had left one cookie, I had to laugh. Did she think that made it okay? But then I stopped laughing because I remembered that chocolate can be poisonous to dogs, and I felt worried.

    I immediately called the vet, who told me to take a turkey baster and squirt hydrogen peroxide down her throat. I locked her in the kitchen while I waited nervously to see if she would throw up. She did. I thought with some amusement, "Good thing she tossed her cookies!"

- When you talk about a difficult experience that you shared as a family—like the death of a grandparent or a pet, or a child's illness, an accident, or a move to a new house—try to give explanations for your and others' negative emotions. "It was especially sad for you that Grandma went into the hospital on Christmas Eve; a time that you expected to be so happy was suddenly scary." Try to talk specifically. "I was scared when you were in the hospital" rather than "it was a difficult time for us."

- When your child tells a story, you can ask how he feels at different points, although asking this too often will make you sound like a therapist, which, even if you are one, doesn't always result in more sharing of feelings. (In fact, I can attest to the fact that it can have the opposite effect.) You could also suggest a feeling. "You sound pretty happy about sitting with Sarah at lunch today."

STORIES WITH A LESSON

We choose to tell some stories because they're entertaining, and others became they make us proud to be part of our family. Another kind of story contains a lesson or a moral. That kind of point goes down much more smoothly in a story than when stating the lesson directly to your child. When I was a young child, my mother made up a story with a lesson for me (stop being such a picky eater because you're really missing out on a lot of great foods), and the moral wasn't lost on me.

The story was this: Susie doesn't like to eat anything but grilled cheese sandwiches for dinner. Walking home each night from the bus with her mother, they look through a neighbor's window and see what's for dinner. One night it's spaghetti and meatballs. The mother thinks it looks delicious and offers to make it for Susie. "Oh no," Susie exclaims. "I won't eat worms and rocks."

When they get home, the mother makes it anyway and puts it down at Susie's place. Susie says, "Eww," and then the phone rings, and the mother leaves the table for a few minutes. When she returns, Susie has eaten everything on her plate, but the mother doesn't say a word about this. The next day, on their walk home, they spy a family eating hamburgers. Susie exclaims, "I'd never eat a brick covered in cement." Again, her mother makes it. Susie initially refuses it and then eats it when her mother isn't looking. This process is repeated over and over until Susie has become an adventurous eater and mother no longer needs to coerce her.

As a picky, timid eater, I was intrigued by this story and asked to hear it over and over. My mother had created a story that put the child in charge of her own eating and gave the mother the role of presenting interesting and appetizing options. The lesson was clear: Mother knew best that her daughter would enjoy many more foods than she was trying.

THE BENEFITS OF STORYTELLING FOR OLDER CHILDREN

It can be a lot of fun for kids to hear tales of their parents' childhood mischief, of grandparents' heroism, of aunts and uncles triumphing over adversity, and of anyone's getting through life's rough patches. These stories can amuse, inspire, and expand for children the repertoire of what it's possible to accomplish in life.

Stories told around the table may be the best way to build resilience and foster optimism in children. Researchers at Emory University's Center for Myth and Ritual found that kids who know more about their family histories suffered less from anxiety and depression and had higher self-esteem. They also had more of a sense of being in charge of their own lives, rather than feeling that things just happened to them.[11]

What might explain the power of family stories to confer these benefits? There's no checklist of family stories that kids need to know to make them more resilient. Is the important ingredient the knowledge of more facts about their families? No, the real connection between family stories and mental health benefits is that in order to learn these stories, children live in families who value sitting down together and listening to one another without distraction. Moreover, what makes family stories so powerful is that they transmit the idea to children that they are part of something bigger than themselves—and their identity enlarges to include the lives of previous generations. Having an "intergenerational self" expands the universe of stories that can inspire dreams or hint at different possibilities that one's own limited life experience doesn't yet contain.

The following example is from a family I saw in therapy: A nine-year-old boy with dyslexia felt frightened, confused, and ashamed when his parents told him at the end of the school year that he would not be returning to his public school next year. Instead, he would attend a special school for kids with learning disabilities.

A few weeks later, during a Fourth of July dinner with the extended family, his grandparents told him that one of his aunts had attended the same school. They told him that before their daughter attended this school, they mistakenly thought that she had very limited intelligence and believed she would have to live with them as an adult. But, at the school, she discovered she loved math, and she went on to become a computer programmer. This story hadn't been told in years. It came to mind because the grandparents saw a helpful connection between their daughter's learning struggles and their grandson's. This story, like others that are almost forgotten, can be brought into the light, shined up and treasured, like a dusty gem found in the attic.

STORIES ABOUT TRAUMA, TRAGEDY, AND TRANSGRESSIONS

No one has a pristine passel of stories to tell. You don't get to be the age of a parent without making some terrible choices or regrettable mistakes along the way. And, as a family therapist, I've rarely met a family that doesn't have a few skeletons rattling around in the closet. Figuring out which stories to tell, which to leave out, and which to clean up before telling presents a real challenge. But leaving out important stories of your family's history also presents a problem, because secrets have tremendous power.

One middle-aged father in my practice didn't want his kids to know that he had been an alcoholic a decade earlier, but he was forced to tell them when a neighbor spilled the beans. One adoptive adolescent didn't speak to her parents for weeks after learning that she had two biological siblings. A mother decided to tell her young adult daughter that she had been sexually abused by a sibling, but the daughter had overheard conversations about the abuse years earlier and had remained painfully silent.

Even when kids don't overhear a conversation, they often sense that there is something they aren't being told. Then, in an effort to make sense of a mysterious vacuum, they will often fill it in—sometimes creating a story that's even worse than the truth. Children who live in families where there are secrets often grow up with the belief that there are things too terrible to speak about. This can be a real burden. But telling these difficult stories at a family dinner can be an incredibly difficult thing to do, and many parents don't want to share these stories at dinner, in the car, before bedtime, not ever.

If you do decide to tell your kids the truth about smoking pot as a teenager, or that you were married before, or that their grandparents had to declare bankruptcy during the Depression, there are a few guidelines that might be helpful.

First, the timing of telling depends largely on the age and maturity of your child, which only you can evaluate. In general, I would never recommend telling a child younger than twelve an upsetting story about her parent's childhood.

Often, the timing is determined by the intersection of something going on now in your child's life and something that happened at a similar time in your own life. When a teenager asks a parent, "Did you ever smoke pot?," answering this question honestly might be dictated by cultural ideas about parents sharing personal transgressions. Some parents may feel that sharing their own missteps will grant their children permission to emulate them. Other parents may feel that sharing such stories will create greater closeness with a teen by putting the parent and child on more equal footing.

In one study, both parents and teens rated highly certain kinds of stories about parents' teenage experimentation with pot: The stories were marked by parents' honesty, their urging of safe experimentation on the part of their teens, their knowledge about marijuana, and their mentioning some regret about their own past experimentation.[12]

It's not just the decisions you make about the timing of telling a story, but it's also important *how* you tell difficult stories. Stories about traumatic events can demonstrate resourcefulness and ways that a relative overcame adversity. Take Justice Sonia Sotomayor's memoir *My Beloved World,* in which she describes the difficulty of receiving a diabetes diagnosis at age seven, while living with an alcoholic father and a mother so angry at her husband that she stayed away from home as much as possible.[13] Justice Sotomayor could have told this story as tragedy, with one terrible thing piling on top of the next. Instead, she recalled a life lesson she learned as a young child that has helped her ever since. She realized that without parents around to help, she had to take over her own diabetes care. In this act of precocious self-reliance, she began to develop the determination and self-discipline that springboarded her later success.

Like Sotomayor, when parents tell painful stories, they might try to weave into the telling a lesson they learned or something good that came out of their challenges. In my family, one of the most common punch lines to a story was a quote from my mother's childhood friend's grandfather: "You never know when your bad luck is your good luck."

Parents

Telling stories about bad luck turning into something good is beneficial for adult storytellers as well as for kids. In a recent study, adults who told such stories showed higher levels of well-being.[14] In fact, adults who tell stories in which suffering leads to growth tend to be more generative or more interested in passing on a positive legacy to the next generation. After all, stories become a kind of keepsake, or part of the legacy that older people want to leave for the next generations.

Regardless of the age of the storyteller, when people are asked to remember events in their past, they are most likely to recall those that occurred when they were late adolescents or young adults. In one study, twenty subjects per decade from teenagers to nonagenarians chose to describe events that took place when they were between the ages of fifteen and thirty-five. These stories also had common themes, mostly about losses or about meeting a personal challenge that resulted in feeling proud of one's achievement.[15] This finding isn't surprising, given the overrepresentation of novels and films about teenagers and young adults. This part of the life cycle seems to capture our imagination regardless of our age, perhaps because this stage is one when we are in the process of becoming someone, a process that continues to unfold throughout our lives.

Older adults tell distinctive stories, according to research that asked young, middle-aged, and older adults to select two stories—one that taught a value and another that taught honesty.[16] The older adults (over sixty years old) were more likely to tell stories with generative and re-demptive themes that were judged to be the most interesting and engag-ing overall. Generative stories are those focused on special opportunities or early blessings of childhood that made the storyteller want to give back later in life. Redemptive themes are ones in which a negative event gets transformed into something positive, usually due to the kindness or gener-osity of another person. People who tell these lemonade-from-lemons, or silk-purse-from- a-sow's-ear type of stories, scored higher on a measure of psychological well-being.[17]

Another feature of stories told by older people, like grandparents, is that the stories are often historical, anchored in the World War II, for example, or the Civil Rights movement. My father delighted in telling his grandsons about attending a Memorial Day parade as a young boy. At that parade, my father saw Civil War veterans who themselves had seen veterans from the Revolutionary War at parades of yesteryear. "This is such a young country," he would observe with a tone of awe. Our families are repositories for our collective history as Americans.

GETTING THE BALL ROLLING WITH STORYTELLING

Sometimes, we need great questions to tell interesting stories. Some won-derful questions are available at Story Corps, the national oral history project that invites Americans to record, share, and preserve stories of their lives. This project honors the importance of everyone's life story. The Story Corps website (www.storycorps.org) contains dozens of questions to inspire storytelling on a wide range of topics, including love, school, work, serious illness, and war. Here are some that kids may want to ask their parents:

- How did you choose my name?
- What was I like as a baby? As a young child?

- Do you remember any of the songs you used to sing to me?
- Who has been the most important person in your life? Can you tell me about him or her?
- What is your earliest memory?
- Where are your mom's and dad's families from?
- Tell me about a grandparent, aunt, uncle, or other relative whom I've never met. What did that person mean to you?
- How has life been different than what you imagined when you were my age?

RECIPE AS STORY

If some of these questions seem a bit too intense for a random Wednesday night dinner, you can let the food spur a story or two. Try telling a story about a food you are eating or about eating a similar food when you were growing up.

Some recipes have a real narrative arc. Here is one of my favorite recipe stories because, when I make this dish for my family, it connects me to the best teacher I've ever had and to my favorite food writer. It's just a sauce, but when I make it and tell the story behind it, I always feel like I'm having a special dinner party.

The recipe and the story start at the table of my beloved English teacher, Frances Taliaferro, and her husband, Lee, who have hosted my family for Fourth of July dinners at their house in Cornwall, Connecticut. We began by reading the Declaration of Independence, and then gathered around a table illuminated by actual candles resting in a dangling chandelier. Franny served the same holiday menu year after year—potato salad, a green salad, baked salmon with a spectacular green sauce, and angel food cake with vanilla yogurt, doused with raspberries she picked herself.

I knew I wanted that green sauce recipe as soon as I tasted it. The recipe—actually it's more of a list of ingredients—comes from Franny's good friend, the deceased writer Laurie Colwin, whose books on home cooking I have read countless times.[18] Here is Franny's story about the green sauce:

"I first became aware of green sauce at Laurie Colwin's table," she said. "She made it at the drop of a hat and served it with all sorts of things. I loved it because it added interest to plain foods, so I asked her for the recipe."

"Oh you just put in whatever you have in the house and whirl it around in the Cuisinart," Laurie said.

"At that point I didn't have much confidence in myself as an improviser, so I asked her to write down the ingredients," Franny said. "This she did, on the nearest note pad, which happened to have a picture of a bear at the top. When Laurie died, I had her 'recipe' framed; it hangs in our kitchen in Cornwall and thus Laurie presides as the Muse of my kitchen.

"So I began experimenting," said Franny, "and discovered that she was absolutely right about putting in whatever you have in the house. The only rule is that the greens must be fresh. In the summer, we grow basil, tarragon, arugula, and parsley. I often have cilantro in the house, sometimes dill. I throw them all in together and don't worry about matching! Watercress is great, but just the stems because the leaves don't add much. I adore capers, in general, and put them in all sorts of things. I wouldn't dream of green sauce without them. I also like a squirt of anchovy paste: you get a slightly marine flavor without having to open and waste a whole can of anchovies. You have to experiment until you find the consistency you like best, which will depend on the amount of oil. This green sauce is like pesto, of course, but doesn't have cheese or nuts."

GREEN SAUCE

(Laurie Colwin's recipe, adapted by Frances Taliaferro)

Fresh greens, any combination of watercress stems, basil, arugula,
    tarragon, parsley, cilantro, and dill
Green onions
Black pepper
Olive oil
Lime or lemon juice
Dry mustard

Capers
Garlic
Dijon mustard
Squirt of anchovy paste

Combine all the ingredients in a food processor to form a thick sauce.

OTHER STORY IDEAS

Just as a recipe can evoke a winding tale, there are objects and artifacts lying about that can also prompt an interesting story. You could hold up a photograph from a family vacation, a grandparents' wedding picture, or your baby picture. Or share a ring that belonged to a family member, or a painting that has hung on the dining room wall without anyone knowing who picked it out, why, or where. Look around you. There are surely an infinite number of conversations ready to be brought to the table.

PART THREE

SERVING IT FORWARD

Using Dinner to Make Change in Your Family and Beyond

8

Lessons Learned from
The Family Dinner Project

The Family Dinner Project is a nonprofit initiative dedicated to helping families use dinner as an opportunity to connect with one another through "food, fun, and conversation about things that matter."[1]
Inspired by the scientific research about the benefits demonstrated among
families who eat together, The Family Dinner Project's mission is to make
it easier for more families to reap these benefits.

In 2010, a group of men and women from a variety of backgrounds—all
of whom shared a belief in the power of family dinners—started to meet
monthly. Our professional backgrounds included education, family therapy, research, design, social work, communication, marketing, and food.[2]
Some of us were experienced home cooks, and others served cereal at dinner. We were mothers, fathers, grandparents, and adults without children.
We knew why dinners were important, but we wanted to provide a road
map—how do you get from knowing that family dinner is a good idea to
the daily practice of cooking healthy foods, and then having a good time at
the table?

Of course, we had many beliefs and stories about family dinners from
our childhoods, and from raising our own children. Even so, we wanted to
learn more, and we hoped to learn from a more diverse group of families

than was represented by our little group. So we invited single parents, three-generational families, same-sex parents, stepfamilies, low-, middle-, and high-income families, and families from many different cultural backgrounds to teach us their best tips. Over time, we incorporated many of these ideas into our website, and tested them out with more families at community dinners and parent workshops that we've hosted all over the country. The result of this work has been twofold: We offer free online resources that thousands of families are using to have more and better dinners. And we work with families in person, through community-based programs in schools, colleges, community clinics, afterschool programs, and neighborhood groups.

In this chapter, you'll learn the best practices that we've found for making dinners simpler, more fun, and more interesting. You'll meet some families we've worked with, and learn how these families set goals for themselves and then went about achieving them. You'll read about some of the grassroots organizing we've done and maybe you'll be inspired to host a dinner or workshop in your community. Along the way, you'll find out what we've discovered about the most important ingredients to making change happen.

OUR BEGINNING IDEAS

Behavior change happens in different ways for different families

Making a commitment to having dinner, preparing it, and staying at the table for conversation is a set of behaviors that may need a little tweaking or a total rebooting, depending on the family's own agenda. Regardless of the *amount* of change needed, when it comes to getting on the road to changing behavior, individuals differ in the *kind* of on-ramp they prefer. Some of us get motivated by *emotion*. We feel in our gut that family dinners are important; we love cooking a delicious meal and having our loved ones eating and talking together. Once we've gotten a taste of that feeling, that's all we need to keep on with family dinners.

Others get going on a new plan through *thinking*—because the benefits of family dinner, documented by research, make logical sense to us, we feel compelled to set a regular family dinner plan in motion.

Still others form new routines by making step-by-step *behavioral* changes. Committing to a program, setting goals, being accountable, and tracking one's progress are essential to creating regular family dinners.

At The Family Dinner Project, we've tried to incorporate each path—emotional, cognitive, and behavioral—as an entry point to change. Regardless of the entry point, we hear from all kinds of families that one of the most powerful parts of The Family Dinner Project is that when they sign up to participate, they join a community of families. For many people, being part of something bigger than themselves is the key to change.

Families know best what goals are important to them

Another important idea: Families need to set their own agendas for change. While the scientific research on family dinners sets five nights a week as the gold standard, real families aren't research subjects. Instead, it's more important that families make the changes in their dinner habits that are meaningful to them. Some families set a goal of having dinner twice a week, while others are already having dinner every night of the week but want to have more fun at the table. Still others want the work of shopping, planning a menu, cooking, serving, and cleaning up to feel more equitable.

We meet families where they are. By asking each family member what he or she would like to improve, we also begin to shift the focus from a parent in charge to everyone feeling a sense of agency. So, let's start with where you are, and where you'd like to be. The goal sheet we give to families who sign up online or who work with us in person is shown in the box on page 142.

Parents are innovators

At The Family Dinner Project, we believe that in any community, parents—not professionals or our team members—are each other's best advisors. If families are the real experts on how to make dinners better, then our job is to get families talking together and sharing the best practices that we've learned in meeting with families all over the country. When we ask families about their dinner challenges, we tend to hear the same ones regardless of

GOAL SHEET

For the following items, please circle a rating from 1 (not at all satisfactory) to 7 (nearly perfect) for where you are now with your dinners. Then do it again, circling the items that are important for you to improve over the next three months. Feel free to leave blank the ones that you are fully satisfied with or that are not important to you.

FOOD

Plan meals in advance	1 2 3 4 5 6 7
Have fun preparing food together	1 2 3 4 5 6 7
Eat nutritious food	1 2 3 4 5 6 7
Try new foods	1 2 3 4 5 6 7
Share the workload	1 2 3 4 5 6 7

FUN

Create a fun, inviting atmosphere	1 2 3 4 5 6 7
Reduce distractions	1 2 3 4 5 6 7
Tell funny stories and laugh together	1 2 3 4 5 6 7
Play games at the table	1 2 3 4 5 6 7

CONVERSATION

Learn about each other's day	1 2 3 4 5 6 7
Make sure that everyone has a voice at the table	1 2 3 4 5 6 7
Talk about things that matter	1 2 3 4 5 6 7
Talk about the kind of people we want to be	1 2 3 4 5 6 7
Discuss the news, books, or movies	1 2 3 4 5 6 7

Try asking the rest of your family to fill this out. Then you can see if there are any shared goals, which will make it easier to work on them together. Another idea is to have each family member fill this out separately, and then play a game: See if you can each guess which are the other's top three goals. This might get everyone engaged in talking about what is most important to improve and why. The point of either of these strategies is to get everyone in your family involved, because this makes everyone an active player and takes the burden off of any one person to make change happen.

the community—not enough time to cook, family members who won't try new foods, a tight budget, conflict at the table, and busy schedules that interfere with the dinner hour. While the challenges are often the same, the solutions that families come up with are creative, novel, and specific.

Dinner is about more than food, though food brings us to the table

Food is usually the gateway to better dinner rituals. Often, when parents start with a focus on improving the food, they find that other parts of the dinner start to change, like the liveliness of the conversation.

WHAT WE LEARNED FROM OUR FIRST PILOT FAMILIES

When we first started The Family Dinner Project, we relied on our own experiences with and our research about family dinners to build a library of tips and resources that we posted on our website. We hoped that these ideas would help other families improve their dinner rituals, but we weren't sure. So we decided to "road test" the ideas with fifteen families that made a commitment to having at least three meals over the course of three months. To learn what was and wasn't helpful, we interviewed these families in depth before, during, and after their participation. As part of this pilot, we hosted our first community dinner event with several of these families, where we cooked together, played games, and tried out conversation starters. We learned a tremendous amount from these early participants about what challenges families faced, what helped, and what was realistic to expect from our online program. Two families who gave us a lot of helpful feedback and insight were the Walkers and the Smith-Bells.

Vanessa and Anthony Walker[3] are parents to three teenagers living at home and four more who have already left home. Anthony contacted The Family Dinner Project because he was afraid that he was losing touch with his kids. Most nights, he told us, his teenagers bought fast food and ate it while holed up in their bedrooms, watching TV. Finances were tight and the parents struggled to put food on the table. Anthony is disabled and was no longer able to work his job as a professional cook. Vanessa worked during the day and went to nursing school at night, so scheduling family dinners was a challenge, too.

The Walkers' goals were to have family dinner together at least once a week, and to have more fun. The parents' first step was to announce to their family that there was going to be a new game plan: They would start eating dinner together. And it would be a home-cooked meal, not Styrofoam boxes with chicken nuggets from a fast-food joint. At first, the kids bellyached and protested. But after a few family dinners things changed.

"They kind of anticipate it," Anthony explained. "They know it's going to be all right. It's going to be a little fun."

As often happens, one change led to another, so that where they ended up wasn't where they expected to be.

The Walker parents got things moving by announcing their commitment to family dinner. Other changes soon followed. The parents found ways to get the children excited about dinner. For one meal, each child picked an ingredient—noodles, broccoli, and meatballs—and voilà! A new recipe was created. They also began to make up games at the table. One game, called Thumbs Up to the Chef, involved grading the chef on taste, presentation, and atmosphere. Anthony got the family talking about current events using "old-school verses, new-school rap," another Walker-invented game. The kids named a current song about something happening in the world right now, and the parents countered with an old song. Vanessa explained further: "By doing this, we can find out how much things have changed and how much they've stayed the same over the years."

After three months, the family that had begun without even a table, and with only an expectation of getting the family together for dinner, got more than it bargained for.

"We got back some of what was lost in the family," Anthony explained. "Sitting down together, talking, and laughing helped us get back a sense of closeness and family unity."

The Smith-Bells,[4] composed of two mothers, a five-year-old son, and one-year-old twin boys, were already eating home-cooked meals together most nights of the week and participating in an organic farm share. Unlike the Walkers, who had just wanted to get the family to sit down for at least one meal a week, the Smith-Bells' goals were to make the work of food preparation more equitable and to make dinner feel like a strong tradition.

When they started with The Family Dinner Project, Monica complained that most of the cooking fell to her because Nora had more pressing work demands. This imbalance led to tensions between the couple. The first change they made was to prepare more meals in advance on the weekends, when everyone could join in. Even the twins looked on and played with eggbeaters. And five-year-old Connor played an active role in cooking.

In order to make dinner feel more like a tradition, they saved big news to share at dinner. The mothers wanted to make sure that everyone had a fair share in the conversation, as well as with the workload. Nora knew that she was charting new territory that hadn't been part of her childhood dinners.

"My parents monopolized the dinner-time conversation, and this is one thing that I didn't want to repeat," she said. So they developed the practice of lighting a candle that gets passed around the table. When a family member holds the candle, it is his or her turn to talk. The candle not only introduced a way to keep the conversation moving, it introduced a symbol that contributed to making dinner feel special, and like more of a ritual.

As with the Walkers, the Smith-Bells exceeded the goals they'd set for themselves. The initial goal of getting the kids more involved in food preparation led to some surprising and unexpected benefits. One night when Monica was preparing acorn squash with Connor, he asked, "How come it's green on the outside and orange on the inside?" This led to a lively discussion about other things in life that aren't always what they seem to be. Including Connor in preparing the meal created an opportunity to discuss a valuable life lesson—you can't judge a book by its cover or a vegetable by its skin color. Dinner turned out to be a place to talk about everyday ethics.

WORKING ON THE GROUND WITH FAMILIES

The Family Dinner Project has worked with communities all over the country in an effort to share ideas about family dinners, to try out the efficacy of our tips with diverse groups of parents and grandparents, and to learn new tips and recipes from others.

Community dinners

After a year of working with families like the Smith-Bells and the Walkers, The Family Dinner Project began hosting regular community dinners in schools, diners, community centers, college cafeterias, and church halls. Not only did parents and their children attend these dinners but also leaders in the community—parent educators, health clinic nutritionists, clergy, afterschool staff, and teachers—so that they could test-drive our materials and ideas and then use them with the families they work with.

The Family Dinner Project partners set up community dinners for many reasons. A middle school in Cumming, Georgia, used a community dinner to get parents talking about becoming more engaged in school, and for kicking off a parent-supported program about improving literacy. At one community dinner in Red Bank, New Jersey, following the devastating Hurricane Sandy, kids made place mats and sent them to kids in Watertown, Massachusetts, who were having a community dinner; then the Watertown kids returned the favor with a delivery of place mats. The message was clear: Another community is thinking about you and cares about the same things that you do.

At a small college in Vermont, where most students are the first in their families to attend college, we organized a community dinner so that students could talk about the importance of college to local high school kids and their parents, many of who had not attended college. And, in West Concord, Minnesota, the goal of a community dinner was to promote health education in a rural county.

Omar's Café

West Concord is about a half hour outside of Rochester, Minnesota (home to the Mayo Clinic). You get there by traveling on Route 14, past farms and grain silos, then down a narrow dirt and gravel road. West Concord has fewer than 800 people, but Omar's Café is a watering hole that attracts diners from all over Dodge County. The sign on the door reads: "Home cooking at its best," with a retro menu of comfort foods like goulash, chili, and beef noodle soup.

On a warm autumn night in 2012, The Family Dinner Project was invited by the Mayo Clinic Center for Innovation to host a community dinner at Omar's Café. About eight families piled in, each occupying a booth with banquettes.

The Mayo Clinic Center for Innovation's reason for this invitation was to be part of their Community Health Transformation initiative, a wide-reaching plan to introduce a new model of healthcare. The clinic was experimenting with ways to improve health and wellness through a number of innovative practices, including increased community engagement outside of the hospital setting. The aim of the partnership with The Family Dinner Project was to bring people together and showcase the long-term positive benefits of family dinners. The ultimate goal was to transform the experience and delivery of healthcare, and at Omar's Café that goal started with fajitas.

As families moseyed in after work, they passed tubs of ingredients, ready for assemblage—sautéed vegetables, grated cheese, olives, salsa, hot sauce, and beans. There were about twenty-five participants from all over Dodge County, with children ranging in ages from five to eighteen. There was an elderly couple, too, who worked at a local food pantry. Omar, the café's longtime owner, remarked that he had never seen such a diverse group of people assembled there before—old and young, low-income and professionals, Latino and Caucasian families.

This dinner event was planned with a structure that mirrored a dinner that families could have at home: Over the course of ninety minutes, participants would cook, talk, and play together. But first we engaged the children as soon as they entered, hoping to tame some end-of-the-day-energy with an invitation to make place mats and to pound on dough to make rolls in the shapes of animals and people. Once each table had place mats and the rolls were ready for baking, we introduced the rationale of the evening—to discuss the emotional, nutritional, and intellectual benefits of family dinner, and to invite this group to share its best practices about how to make dinner happen despite busy schedules and tight budgets.

The families didn't know one another, so we suggested a quick ice-breaker. Each person said his or her name, a favorite family meal, and a favorite thing to do together as a family. Then we plunged into making dinner together. Each table was equipped with a few avocados, a lemon, sour cream, salsa, and garlic so that each family could mash the avocados to create guacamole. With the appetizers done and the rolls hot, each participant took a tortilla and customized fillings for it, choosing among the variety of ingredients laid out.

After everyone had made a couple of fajitas, we suggested a conversation for each family to have over dinner. We asked the children to interview their parents about what dinner was like when the parents were children. These were some suggested questions that kids could ask their parents:

- What was your favorite food when you were a child?
- Who sat where? Can you draw a picture of your childhood dinner table? Did you have a special seat as a child? If so, how was it chosen, and what do you think the seating arrangements convey?
- Who decided the menu? What did you do if there were differences in food preferences? Did kids or parents decide? Were there compromises, turn taking, or multiple meals made?
- Who shopped, cooked, served, and cleaned up?
- What did you talk about at dinner?
- What do you most want to carry forward or leave behind from those experiences?

After dinner, we asked if anyone wanted to share a story of childhood dinners.

(These questions tend to provide a snapshot of what a childhood was like. So when we reminisce about childhood dinners we are also remembering what was bitter and sweet, sour and salty about our relationships with our parents and siblings. Not every dinner memory is going to be a happy one. But parents don't need to rely solely on their childhood experiences to build a vibrant dinner practice with their children. Our hope is The Family Dinner Project provides enough resources and ideas to kick-start a commitment to family dinners, even if parents recall their childhood dinner tables with ambivalence.)

When it was time for dessert, the children traipsed off with a few members of our team. Once outdoors, they poured heavy cream into plastic containers. Then they shook the living daylights out of these tubs, passing them from child to child while dancing to music until the liquid cream became whipped cream that could be dolloped onto apple crisp. The children plated up the desserts and served them to their parents, who had been having a conversation about their biggest dinnertime challenges.

Stephanie, a mother of two young children with a husband in school, confided that she was overwhelmed by balancing three different school schedules on top of her own work schedule. Other parents offered their solutions to similar scheduling challenges. Stephanie came away from this dinner with a new idea of a weekly meal planner, suggested by another busy parent, as a way to make the most of limited time available.

During dessert, we suggested the game Two Truths and a Tall Tale (described in Chapter 6). This game is one of many on our website that families can try to make dinner more fun, and so to keep kids at the table longer.

At the very end of the evening, we told the families about The Family Dinner Project's "Food, Fun and Conversation: 4 Weeks to Better Family Dinners," which is packed with ideas and resources that we have collected from families all over the country. We asked them to try it in their own homes and then to gather again at Omar's Café in a month's time to share their experiences.

The structure of this family dinner has been repeated at community dinners across the country. You can try it, too, at your local elementary school, religious hall, or any other place where your community gathers. It starts with an activity for kids to do when they first arrive, followed by an icebreaker so that everyone gets a chance to say hello. There's an opportunity to cook together, and then while eating, families are invited to try having a conversation that's different from the customary "How was your day?"

Next, the children go off with a team member to make dessert so that parents have a few minutes to talk about their own dinner challenges and solutions. Once dessert is served, the families are taught a game to play. At the end of the dinner, families learn about our four–week program, which can extend and expand the experience they have just had. They're asked to return in a month and share what the experience was like.

THE FAMILY DINNER PROJECT'S FAJITAS (FOR 24)

6 red onions, thickly sliced

12 bell peppers (red, green, or combination), seeded and sliced into strips

2 tablespoons minced garlic

6 yellow squash, halved and sliced into strips

Vegetable oil

3 cups salsa

2 tablespoons ground cumin

3 teaspoons salt

8 (15-ounce) cans black beans, rinsed

48 (8-inch) flour tortillas

6 cups shredded cheddar cheese

1½ cups chopped fresh cilantro

Sauté the onions, peppers, garlic, and squash in vegetable oil in a large frying pan over medium heat for about 10 minutes. In a separate pan, heat the salsa, cumin, and salt for about 5 minutes.

Wrap the tortillas in foil, and heat them in a 350-degree oven for about 15 minutes. Give each participant two tortillas, and let them fill each one by spooning ingredients evenly down the center of the tortilla. Each person can choose among several options to stuff their tortilla—vegetable mixture, salsa, cheese, and cilantro—or choose them all. Roll up the tortillas, and enjoy.

WHIPPED CREAM WITH BERRIES

4 pints cold whipping cream

Fresh berries or other fruit

Using a plastic container with a tight-fitting lid, fill it halfway (or less) with whipping cream. Put the lid on tightly, and shake, shake, shake! You can pass the container from person to person and encourage jumping, running, singing, dancing, and rolling on the floor while keeping the container tightly closed. Be sure to check after a couple of minutes because if you go too far, you'll end up with butter.

Dollop some of the whipped cream on sliced berries.

Parent and grandparent workshops

In addition to community dinners, our organization also facilitates parent and grandparent workshops, where only one adult attends, rather than a whole family. This format allows for a smaller group that can potentially reach a greater number of families. For example, we can easily host fifteen adults in a workshop, whereas if those same adults brought along their families, we would have a boisterous group of more than sixty people.

The workshops are usually offered in a package of two. The first focuses on the challenges and solutions to creating a family dinner ritual, relying on the expertise in the group to solve common problems. The second workshop is about learning how to make the most of conversation at the dinner table—interesting conversation starters, ways to deepen the conversation once it starts, suggestions for different types of storytelling, and games to play.

In an after-school community building in Lynn, Massachusetts, ten grandmothers gathered around primary-color rectangular tables to talk about family dinners. This meeting was part of an ongoing weekly gathering of a state-run group for women who are raising their grandchildren. The following week they planned to talk about bringing out the best in their grandchildren. For two hours with us, they compared the obstacles they confronted in getting their families together each night to enjoy a home-cooked meal. Then they brainstormed solutions.

Three members of The Family Dinner Project were along to conduct a workshop we have taken on the road many times before. We started with a check-in or icebreaker so that everyone had a chance to speak about the way family, memory, culture, and food are intermingled like a well-simmered stew. We asked the women, "What is a food memory you have from your family growing up?" Almost everyone offered a memory tied to a special holiday dish, and all the memories were positive ones. Cleo rhapsodized about an Easter treat of sweet beans, milk, and sugar from her home country, the Dominican Republic. It was a dish her grandmother taught her to make. Paula, an African-American woman, described the collard greens and cornbread that "you *have* to have for any family gathering." And Pat, a Polish woman, shared her memories of Christmas Eve dinners of beet soup and fish. John Sarrouf, a team member of The Family Dinner Project, who was leading the discussion, commented, "Traditions help us all feel like we belong to something."

The goal of the meeting was to ask about the challenges these women face at dinnertime and then harness their collective wisdom to generate solutions. I started by asking about what is often the most difficult challenge for any of us: What do you do well? Using a flip chart, Grace, another team member, wrote down the strengths that the grandmothers offered:

- I make time for everybody to sit down together.
- I help create meaningful conversation.
- My grandchildren feel heard and valued.
- I make a delicious soup that brings everyone to the table.
- I like to make new foods.
- I can cook a meal in forty-five minutes or less.
- My grandchildren want to help or want to learn how to cook.

We then asked about the obstacles to making dinner and keeping everyone engaged. Most of the challenges were variations on the same two themes: the struggle to expand children's food choices so that the grandmothers aren't cooking the same meal night after night (or cooking multiple meals to accommodate disparate tastes), and the problem of limited time for cooking given competing responsibilities of work and childcare.

"As wise grandparents, you have all the creativity and skills right here in this group to share with one another in order to solve these challenges,"

John explained. The challenges tend to be same at every workshop—not enough time or money, family members who won't eat the same meal, parents who don't like to cook, too much nagging at the table.

The group brainstormed ideas to meet the common challenges. In thinking about how to expand children's food choices, for example, they generated many useful ideas:

- Blend vegetables into a soup to get kids to eat more variety.
- Substitute a fruit for a vegetable, like roast chicken with apples, instead of with carrots.
- Make dinner special by setting the table and lighting a candle.
- Use leftovers to make an interesting new meal. One woman, from the Dominican Republic, offered her recipe for empanadas, which is a great way of reusing food from the night before (see the recipe that follows).
- Involve kids by getting them to help with cooking or shopping.
- Serve raw vegetables for kids to munch on while you're cooking.
- Put one new ingredient alongside something they already like.

EMPANADAS FROM CLEO

Leftover meat

Leftover vegetables

Guava, peeled, seeded, and chopped

Cream cheese

A stack of disc pastries (find discs in the frozen foods section of the supermarket)

Canola oil (optional)

Add leftover meat, vegetables, or a combination of guava and cream cheese to the center of a pastry disc. Fold the pastry over and seal the edges with a fork or using your fingers.

Fry the discs in canola oil, or place them on a baking sheet and bake in a 350-degree oven for about 10 minutes.

John mentioned an idea he learned from a parent at another workshop: Instead of asking a child to take a *bite* of a new food, ask him to take a *taste*, and then describe it. Paying attention to the taste slows down a child's quick rush to judgment about a new food. This solution isn't found in textbooks. Rather, it is an example of one parent's wisdom passed from one community to another.

After the discussion of common challenges and unique solutions, the women moved into the kitchen, where Grace had assembled all the ingredients needed to make lasagna. The grandmothers would take the dish home and serve it for dinner or freeze it for another busy night.

Despite the extra challenges these women faced—strained relationships with the parents of their grandchildren, declining health, and limited budgets—they were eager to try new things to improve family dinners. They agreed to try The Family Dinner Project's four-week program and meet again in a month for another workshop. At this second session, they planned to share their experiences with the "4 Weeks to Better Family Dinner" program, and also focus on making the most of conversation at the table. Many of the grandmothers exchanged recipes as they headed out the door, lasagna pan in tow.

THE FAMILY DINNER PROJECT'S EASY LASAGNA

15 ounces ricotta cheese

2 large eggs

½ cup Parmesan cheese, shredded

4 cups shredded mozzarella cheese, divided

¼ teaspoon salt

¼ teaspoon pepper

2 tablespoons chopped fresh basil (optional)

3 garlic cloves, minced (optional)

1 (45-ounce) can tomato-and-basil pasta sauce

8 ounces no-boil lasagna noodles

3 cups fresh baby spinach

Preheat the oven to 375 degrees. Grease a 13- × 9-inch baking pan.

Combine the ricotta cheese, eggs, Parmesan cheese, ½ cup of the mozzarella cheese, salt, pepper, basil, and garlic in a bowl.

Spread about 1 cup of the tomato sauce at the bottom of the greased pan.

Arrange a layer of lasagna noodles on top (about four noodles will cover the pan). It's fine if they overlap.

Next, layer ⅓ cup of the ricotta cheese mixture, one-third of the spinach (it will shrink, don't worry), 1 cup of the mozzarella cheese, and about 1 cup pasta sauce.

Repeat the layering twice more in this order: noodles, ricotta mixture, spinach, mozzarella, and sauce. On top layer noodles, the remaining sauce, and the remaining mozzarella.

Cover with aluminum foil, and bake 40 to 50 minutes. Remove the foil and bake 5 minutes longer to brown the cheese on top. Let stand 5 minutes before serving.

DO-IT-YOURSELF DINNER PARTIES

After participating in community dinners and parent workshops, several families asked us, "What's next?" In response, we came up with the idea of DIY dinner parties, so that a community of friends could help sustain the practice of family dinners.

You find two other families to share some food, fun, and conversation, and you agree to have three dinners total—one dinner at each family's house over the course of several weeks. Here is a sample plan for a DIY:

Start with an icebreaker: Ask everyone assembled to tell a favorite family meal memory.

Make an appetizer together: Have one family bring the ingredients to make guacamole.

GUACAMOLE

3 avocados, peeled, pitted, and mashed
1 teaspoon salt

3 garlic cloves, minced

1 lime or lemon, juiced

1 pinch cayenne pepper

Crackers or chips

In a medium bowl, mash together the avocados, salt, garlic, and lime juice. Stir in the cayenne pepper.

Serve with crackers or chips.

Make the main course together: Have one family bring the fixings to make pizzas.

PIZZA (FOR 4 FAMILIES)

2 cups marinara sauce, divided

4 (12-inch) premade pizza crusts

1½ cups Parmesan cheese, divided

Additional toppings (allow for about ½ cup per pizza): pepperoni, peppers, mushrooms, olives, broccoli, spinach, pineapple, or onions

Preheat the oven to 450 degrees.

Spread ½ cup of the sauce over each crust, and then sprinkle each with ¼ cup Parmesan cheese. Add other toppings as desired. Sprinkle the remaining cheese over the toppings on each pizza and then bake for about 10 minutes or until the cheese is bubbling.

Toast: Name one thing you're grateful for.

Play a game: Charades or Pictionary are possibilities, or another game of your choice.

Include everyone in a conversation: Everyone says a "rose" (the best part of the day) and a "thorn" (the most difficult part of the day).

Make dessert: Have the third family bring the dessert ingredients.

FRUIT AND YOGURT PARFAITS

Nonfat or low-fat vanilla yogurt

Granola

Fresh or frozen berries (strawberries, blueberries, raspberries,
    blackberries, or a combination)

Honey

Each guest layers yogurt, granola, and fruit into a small bowl or cup, and
then drizzles honey over the top.

Another idea (best in the warm weather) is to text several families or
friends in your neighborhood a few hours before dinner: "Bring your dinner to the beach or to a local park, and we'll all eat together." Again you are
involving your community in the celebration of family dinners.

THE ONLINE PROGRAM: FOUR WEEKS TO BETTER FAMILY
DINNERS

Food, Fun and Conversation: 4 Weeks to Better Family Dinners brings
together many of the ideas we've learned in working with hundreds of
families from all over the country. It's free and available online at thefamily
dinnerproject.org.

For each of four weeks, the family is asked to focus on a different aspect
of family dinner. The first week is all about *making a commitment* to family
dinners and figuring out what your goals are for better dinners. The second
week emphasizes *making it simple*—or figuring out ways to cut down on
the work involved in making dinners. This could include getting everyone
to help, pre-making meals over the weekend, or planning meals a week
ahead so you can be sure to have all your ingredients on hand. The third
week is about *making it fun*. During this week, families are encouraged to
have more fun with cooking and to play games at the table. In week four,
families are asked to *make it matter,* to take advantage of this reliable time
of the day when the family can have a group conversation.

We have tracked the progress of about thirty families who filled out a survey before and after their participation in the four-week program.

Overall, this is what we learned:

- The act of signing up for the project was powerful in helping families start to change behaviors. When families felt that they were part of something that involved other people with similar goals, they felt motivated to set goals and stick to them. As one mother put it: "It's affirming to know that I am part of something, a community."
- A family's initial stated goal did not always correspond with the aspect of dinner about which they reported feeling the greatest increase in satisfaction. For example, families that wanted to work on greater food selection and easier dinner preparation ended up feeling best about their improvements in enjoying one another's company and having fun. Families that wanted to have more fun ended up feeling that they had made the most change in being able to talk about things that matter.
- Nearly every family believed that participating in the four-week program had led to improvements in family dinners.

Since 2010, we've helped thousands of families make the changes they want in their dinnertime rituals: Families start to eat healthy dinners where they used to eat only fast food. A parent burdened by making a different meal for each family member learns to engage everyone in the dinner-making process; lo and behold, as a by-product, she gets everyone to agree on eating the same meal. Parents who have grown weary of asking, and kids who have grown weary of answering the same question night after night, discover many ways to enliven the table conversation.

But it's not only concrete behavioral changes that you can make to your family dinner. You may also want to make some adjustments to repetitive patterns and roles. We'll turn to these issues in the next chapter.

9

Dinner as a Laboratory for Change

'm a huge fan of eating better, having more fun, feeling less burdened by cooking, and getting the conversational juices flowing at the table. But these aren't the only changes that can happen at dinner. As a therapist, I've witnessed other types of transformation occur when families engage in the process of cooking and eating.

A family dinner is like an improvisatory theater performance or a laboratory experiment. The family shows up night after night, and as a group they can try out new ways of interacting with one another. Like actors in a troupe, they can try new behaviors, habits, and roles. A director (or a therapist) can provide a new setup or opening line to an improv, but then the troupe takes it and runs with it. Like scientists in a laboratory, a family can figure out which experiments work better than others. One change in the laboratory can lead to others—some planned and others serendipitous.

Changes in family relationships can happen in two ways. The first is by experimenting with new cooking roles. A couple can work on becoming better collaborators by starting to cook together. Or a teenager who has been critical of everything his parents do might start to make dinner. As he feels more involved and valued as a contributing family member, his contrariness might diminish.

The second way is by trying out new behaviors at the dinner table. For example, one family I worked with complained that there was too much bad-mouthing and name-calling in their exchanges with one another. While we could explore this for an hour in therapy, it was much more powerful to use dinnertime itself as an annex to the family therapy office, an annex they had access to *every* night of the week. With this in mind, the family decided to try an experiment of listening to one another at dinner without saying a critical word. If someone "slipped," family members interrupted to say, "Rephrase that, please!"

In this chapter, you'll read about other families who have used the dinner hour to make relationship changes: reworking power inequities in a couple's relationship; reconnecting an estranged child and parent; getting a do-over as an adult after an abusive childhood; and coming to terms with a new stage of life. These changes all began in therapy but took root at home, where they could be tested night after night, since the dinner table keeps presenting itself as a place to try out new things.

USING COOKING TO MOVE FROM COMPETITION TO COLLABORATION

Rosa and Juan,[1] a middle-aged couple with two teenage daughters, are medical researchers at a teaching hospital. They came to see me for couples therapy when their relationship had morphed from being supportive collaborators at home and at work to becoming resentful competitors and estranged spouses. After months of therapy, a breakthrough occurred when we delved into their cooking practices. To be more precise—a breakthrough occurred during our *second* foray into their cooking practices. The first attempt was pretty much a kitchen disaster, like serving a raw chicken at a dinner party.

First the back story about the couple: For the first twenty years of marriage, Rosa and Juan had been very supportive of one another's work, even coauthoring many scholarly papers. But that changed when Rosa suffered a depression that sapped her powers of concentration and attention. Instead of helping each other navigate the quirks of academic life, Rosa believed that Juan was just out for himself, and Juan, for his part, was angry with

Rosa. He didn't really understand what her depression had to do with her loss of intellectual focus.

Juan, an intense man who was more comfortable arguing a point than asking questions to understand Rosa's perspective, explained their troubles this way: "We fight a lot, but that's not the problem. We were equals, but with Rosa's depression, we're not. I don't know how to be with her any more."

Rosa was no shrinking violet. She had a great capacity to express emotion and to engage Juan in debate on everything from avant-garde French cinema to feminist interpretations of moral development.

After several weeks of therapy they had a shared understanding about Rosa's depression as a real medical condition. But despite this insight, and despite the fact that Rosa's depression was now being treated with medication and individual therapy, they had yet to restore their vibrant relationship as intellectual peers and engaged partners. Instead, Juan withdrew from Rosa and had become more self-reliant. And Rosa, frustrated in her attempt to engage Juan, resorted to provoking him in order to get any response at all.

Although Juan stuck to himself most of the time, he loved to cook for the family, as his father did, and he spent at least an hour each night in the kitchen. He insisted, however, on cooking alone and without a cookbook. He preferred to create recipes out of his imagination or from his memory of childhood meals.

One day, Juan began a therapy session with a cooking question that he wanted to discuss. I felt excited and leaned forward in my chair—this must be how a psychoanalyst feels when a patient offers a dream.

Juan told Rosa that he had been thinking about a dessert that his mother used to make—a frothy meringue swimming in sauce, called a floating island. He asked Rosa if she would make it for him, and she was visibly pleased by his request; Juan hadn't asked her to share the kitchen with him in years, so this invitation had extra heft. Rosa confided that baking and making sauces were the only things she learned to do in the kitchen when she was a child. Most of all, Rosa felt invited into Juan's emotional world after feeling iced out for years. Here in one fell swoop was a chance to enter both his kitchen and the closely guarded chamber of his inner world. However, she overstepped when she asked him why he was thinking about his mother. This was more than Juan bargained for. He rebuked her. "I have no idea," he said. "I'd just like you to make the dessert." Rosa settled for that and agreed to try it that night.

The next week, I contained my curiosity for a few minutes before I blurted out, "How did the dessert turn out?" I could tell by their glum faces that it didn't go well. Rosa's version of a floating island involved beating egg whites and then baking them to form toasted peaks over soft pillows of cream. Juan's childhood confection, however, involved raw eggs and bore no resemblance to Rosa's creation. Rosa, still undaunted, saw these two different takes on meringues as a chance to discuss their different families. But Juan was not interested in sharing these feelings with Rosa. "I just wanted you to make the dessert the way I wanted," he said.

"Juan, you are so controlling," Rosa retorted. "I wanted to play with you and talk with you about your family."

As their therapist, I saw this incident as containing their central conflict: Juan wanted to keep emotion away, and Rosa wanted to bring it in. Juan had been burned by Rosa's emotionality, as he blamed her depression on the breakdown of their marriage. They managed this conflict by trying to vie for control. "Let's do things my way" is what they seem to be saying to each other, to no good effect.

Their different styles had grown rigid and polarized over the years. Juan was wary about letting Rosa in and tried to protect himself by being controlling. Rosa felt frozen out, and when given any opportunity to penetrate Juan's fortress, she overwhelmed him with her emotions. But, if this conflict was bubbling up in the kitchen, perhaps it could be worked on there. I suggested a way to cooperate as fellow chefs that would begin to restore their sense of play and collaboration and wouldn't put either one in charge. Privately, I worried that I might be on shaky ground, given how badly the last cooking episode went. But I pressed on, remembering that the kitchen is the place that Juan feels most generous and expressive.

So, nervously, I wondered out loud if there was a way they could work together in the kitchen so that neither of them was giving or receiving orders. Maria, their eighteen-year-old high school senior, was about to leave home, and Ana, their seventeen-year-old high school junior, would leave in another year, so I suggested that maybe they'd like to teach them some cooking skills. I asked what was most important to teach them.

Juan answered first. "I want them to try new things and take risks."

Rosa added, "To quote the Dalai Lama, I want them to cook and love with reckless abandon."

Their responses made me feel that I could persevere. I suggested that they find a recipe that neither of them had ever made before, cook it, and then teach their daughters how to make it. In that way they would incorporate the value of trying new things. They decided to find a recipe from a Latin culture that is neither Argentinian like Rosa nor Guatemalan like Juan. Instead, they decided to re-create a chicken with a rich *mole* sauce from their favorite Mexican restaurant.

The next week, before I had a chance to ask, they told me that the dish was delicious, although their children gave it mixed reviews. They described the fun they had together figuring out how to make a mole sauce, tinkering with the spices, and creating a recipe all their own. And, as they were leaving my office that morning, Juan tossed off a comment: "Did we mention that we are collaborating on a paper together for the first time in years?"

I don't think the timing of this academic collaboration was a coincidence. Instead, I think that much as children might work out a conflict through playing with stuffed animals, Juan and Rosa began to work out a prickly marital conflict through cooking. The success of collaborating on a new recipe opened the door for collaborating on an intellectual project. This was not a miracle cure. The mole sauce did not lead to marital bliss. It did, however, give them one experience of creative collaboration that I could remind them of when they despaired of ever being able to work together as equals.

USING COOKING TO RECONNECT A FATHER
AND HIS ADOLESCENT SON

In my clinical practice, a family came to see me for help with their seventeen-year-old son, Ben, who was described as oppositional and who had stopped talking to his father, except to ask for a ride to school. The father, Roy, complained to me: "Ben is everything I am not. I am a Republican, so he is an anarchist. I have worked hard to achieve material success, and he has nothing but contempt for my achievements. I am socially conservative, and he has hair down to his shoulders. The last indignity is that he is a vegetarian, and he won't eat our food."

When I asked them about other recent changes in the family, they told me that Mary, Ben's mother, had recently quit her job. As a result, she was doing all the cooking, taking over from Roy, who used to make dinner for the family. Ben piped up, "I wish my mother was still working, since I don't like her cooking."

I ventured to articulate the implied compliment to his father: "So I guess your father's a pretty good cook." Ben nodded and smiled. Encouraged, I continued. "What was dinner like when your father cooked it?"

"I'd keep my dad company while he prepared dinner," Ben answered. "I might make a suggestion—try some chili powder, or go easy on the onions. And he'd usually do it."

"Of course, I would," Roy quickly added. "I was so happy to have your company. Mary and Ben have an easy time talking about movies and books. But this was the one time of the day we would talk."

I ventured a comment to Ben: "Maybe it's not that you object to your mother's cooking, but that you're protesting losing the time with your father."

The father nodded, but added, "I don't think he'd like my cooking now any better than he likes his mother's, since he's become a vegetarian."

A child changing the way he eats during adolescence is a familiar story. An omnivore child becomes a die-hard adolescent vegan. A sweet tooth is traded in for a love of pickled foods. A passion for ice cream becomes so intense that new flavors are invented each week and the ice cream maker is in constant use. Food choices, like decisions about hair color, music, and clothing, are time-honored opportunities for teenagers to differentiate themselves from their parents and to assert that they no longer have the childish tastes of yesteryear. So Ben's recent decision to become a vegetarian didn't sound like a full-scale rejection of his parents. Instead, I noted that Roy and Mary could benefit from eating more vegetables, grains, fruits, and nuts, even if they continued to eat meat. Ben might very well be helping them to live longer.

Even though I thought I might be pressing my luck, I went on to suggest that Roy buy a book on vegetarian cooking and then ask Ben to pick out some particularly good recipes that his father could make a couple of nights a week. In this way, father and son could renew their partnership in the kitchen but with an adjustment to accommodate Ben's shift to vegetarianism. While Roy felt rejected by all the ways that Ben was asserting his autonomy, in the kitchen they could find a way to make room for these changes and for their mutual longing for connection.

Parents engage in many pushes and pulls around adolescents' growing demands for more autonomy and self-definition. When a parent agrees to change the family's foods to make room for a teenager's new tastes, it can go a long way to easing some of these tensions. When Roy agreed to join Ben in his new vegetarian world, it was a way of saying to him, "I'm interested in the person you are becoming." When Ben was willing to pick a recipe for Roy to make, it was a way of saying, "I'm not rejecting you. I just want you to know me differently than you did when I was a child."

YOU DON'T HAVE TO REPEAT THOSE AWFUL CHILDHOOD DINNERS

Making family dinners as an adult can be daunting, especially if dinners as a child were painful and unpleasant. But current family dinners can also provide an opportunity for a second chance.

This was the situation with Nora, who came to individual therapy with a set of childhood wounds that were only barely scarred over but never fully healed. Talking about her dinners growing up identified the wounds; talking about her current family dinners was a place to start the repair.

Nora, a single mother of three young children, came to me for parenting advice. As a way of learning more about her childhood, I asked her to tell me about the family dinners she had while growing up. She winced visibly and then told me straight out that she wasn't ready to talk about them. Since most patients are willing to talk about childhood dinners,

Nora's response concerned me, but I knew that I'd have to wait until she was ready to tell me more.

Months later, we circled back when I noticed that she had been losing weight. She told me that eating was really hard for her, especially when she was having a difficult time managing other parts of her life. She had just been laid off from her job and felt scared that she wouldn't find employment soon enough to stave off a financial crisis. With a reluctant sigh, she said, "Well, I guess it's time to tell you about what food was like in my childhood home."

Nora was one of four children with a mother who came to dinner after drinking wine all day long. To this day, Nora has no idea why she was singled out for the punishment of having to watch her siblings enjoy their dinners while she was served nothing.

This particular abuse haunts her as a mother. She tells me that while she loves cooking dinner for her three children and talking with them while they eat, she cannot eat in front of them. They have begun to notice. As an excuse, she tells them that she tasted so much of the food while she was cooking that she isn't hungry anymore. This may work for now, while her kids are small, but she acknowledges that they will soon start to ask more questions. And so, with some encouragement, she experimented with eating a few bites in front of them. It was difficult but doable. Now she's getting a second chance at the family she didn't have as a child—one bite at a time.

Like Nora, many parents have no sunny memories of family dinners to build on. But that isn't a prerequisite for creating warm and positive family dinners today. The capacity to nurture differently than one was nurtured as a child doesn't give you back a terrific childhood, but it can deflate its power to define you.

USING DINNERS TO HELP MAKE A TRANSITION TO A NEW LIFE STAGE

In general, families and couples are most challenged during the transition from one stage of life to another—the first year of marriage, the adjustment to becoming parents, and much later, becoming "empty nesters." These threshold times stir us up. It's hard work to shed one role and make room for another. Such molting can be a time when our rituals no longer fit us, like a pair of jeans we're beginning to outgrow. If we pay attention to the discomfort, however, rituals such as dinner can be altered to accommodate our new developmental stage. Let's take a look at a few transition points that were difficult and where changing the dinner ritual helped ease the transition.

The-transition-to-marriage dinner debacle

When two people marry, or when they make a long-term commitment to each other, they have dozens of decisions to make. Most broadly, couples at this stage are trying to figure out what they each want to carry forward (and leave behind) from their respective childhoods, and how they will gel their two family experiences: Where will we live? How will we argue? What religion, if any, will we observe? Who will our friends be? Will we go out or stay home on Saturday nights? What will dinnertime be like?

When I ask newly married couples about dinner, the question is a pipeline into their childhoods. Typically, they each describe a complex and compact picture of home life. They can put their two snapshots of childhood family dinners side by side, and they can view the cover to their new family album. Looking at the two pictures side by side, the couple can have this conversation: Now that I see your picture, perhaps I can adjust mine, and vice versa.

Liza and Thomas, a couple who had been married just six months, had a recurring fight about dinner—a fight that made sense only when they examined the dinners of their childhoods. Liza complained that she knocked herself out night after night making four-course gourmet meals for her new husband, and he never even said thank you. She was hurt and angry that Thomas ignored her efforts to please and delight him. Thomas, for his part, said that he hadn't asked for these meals, and if she wanted to make them, he figured that she must enjoy doing so.

When asked to describe their childhood meals, Thomas told of growing up in a family with a single mother who had a degenerative neurological disease but somehow managed to drag herself out of bed each day to make dinner. Every night was the same meal: Spam meatloaf. When his mother would offer him seconds, Thomas remembered biting his tongue so as not to blurt out how repulsive the meal had been, and how he had barely been able to eat firsts, never mind seconds. Instead, so as not to hurt her feelings he would merely say, "I don't need any more tonight."

Liza, the eldest of three, had a mother who died of ovarian cancer when Liza was thirteen. After her mother's death, Liza took over the cooking in the family, making elaborate dinners in order to keep alive the memory of her mother and to create a feeling of home for herself, her younger siblings, and her father.

When she cooked for Thomas, she thought he would understand all the meaning that was packed into the newlywed dinners—the mix of generosity and sacrifice, the connection that ran through her families, from her mother to herself and now to Thomas. But instead of understanding, he was channeling his own sad family dinners. The couple had to unpack these experiences before they were free to create a new dinnertime ritual. While Thomas and Liza had particularly painful family dinners to make sense of, any couple will have two different sets of experiences to integrate into a new interpretation of dinner.

The empty empty-nest dinner table

George and Amy came to see me for couples therapy after their third and last child had left for college. They were finding it difficult to find things to talk about with each other, and they were growing more and more distant. The only time they did talk was to fight about Amy feeling ignored by George, or George feeling unappreciated by Amy.

I asked about dinnertime, which I imagined would be a poignant reminder of their new station in life as empty nesters. George quickly responded in a tone dripping with sarcasm, "If you like three- to four-day-old food served in Tupperware containers, then you'll love dinner at our house. Now, don't get me wrong—every few days, Amy will prepare a hot meal."

Amy listened quietly and then through clenched teeth said, "The table is set before dinner. I feed my husband well, but nothing is ever good enough. George must be living on another planet if he thinks we have left-overs every night."

There was the problem, writ clearly: Without their kids at home, dinner was a time when they keenly felt their disconnection from and disappointment in each other. George believed that Amy didn't want to cook just for him, and Amy felt sure that her efforts to be a good wife were being denigrated. Dinner was a painful nightly reminder of how lost they were without their children.

There were many issues to work on, but their dinner ritual was a time when so much of their unhappiness crystallized. And, because it happened every night, they could try out new behaviors and get quick feedback.

I asked them to consider using dinner as a workshop, to do test runs on interactions that were making them unhappy at the table—and elsewhere. Could they, for example, make a few stabs at offering appreciation at dinner, perhaps about the food, or about some aspect of the other's character, or parenting, or appearance? Could they privately try to notice any goodwill on the part of the other? Perhaps something new would happen if they tried asking for what they wanted at dinner, in terms of food and conversation, rather than trashing what was offered.

Because I believe that it's easier to bear hardships when they are named rather than tucked into dark corners, I suggested that they talk at dinner about missing having the kids at home. But a kid moving out isn't just about loss, so why not also discuss what foods they are freer to eat or what conversations they can have without their kids around. Dinner in bed? A trip they want to plan without the kids? Making spinach crepes that the kids had turned up their noses at?

I won't pretend that these interventions alone made everything hum again for Amy and George. But they did provide a starting point for bridging the gulf between them. Each night, they had a reliable time to reach across the emotional divide that had deepened since their last child moved out. My hope was that by redesigning their dinner ritual, they would begin to find new ways to communicate with each other. One of the great properties of a ritual is that it's set apart from the rest of the day, so it allows for experimentation within borders. Amy and George, like other couples who have lots of problems to solve, can use dinner as a time to try some new ways of being with each other.

FOCUSING ON DINNERTIME TO ADJUST TO OTHER MAJOR DISRUPTIONS IN FAMILY LIFE

Just about every family experiences one or more major disruptions during the children's growing-up years. Common events, such as divorce, remarriage, a parent's illness, a job loss, or a move to a new neighborhood, can generate a seismic shift in day-to-day life, leading to the feeling that the family is inalterably changed. When there has been a major shift in a family, dinner, along with many other routines, gets disrupted too. Making sure that a dinner ritual persists, especially during a time of tumult, is enormously helpful to children. It gives them a sense of stability. Protecting predictable routines and rituals is one of the best things that parents can do for kids, and for themselves, during times of upheaval. And paying attention to changing the dinner ritual to accommodate or honor a major shift can help with the adjustment to a new family configuration.

When parents divorce

In the first year or two following a divorce, most children and parents struggle to get their bearings. Children's routines—eating, homework, bedtime, visiting with friends, going to athletic practices—get disrupted when they're dividing their time between two homes. Dinner can be a particularly poignant time to notice these changes.

For starters, the empty chair of the missing parent is a nightly reminder of the divorce. And despite the best efforts of the single parent who has tried to prepare a nice dinner, mealtime can be a time of deep longing for the parent who isn't there. Children who liked to talk and linger over dinner may want to finish as quickly as possible, to avoid feeling the pain of loss.

Several things might help. Naming a child's sadness, and letting children talk about how different dinner feels now is a good start. If loud conflict, heavy drinking, or violence was the reason for the divorce, children might also note that dinnertime is more peaceful now. They may feel guilty about preferring the divorced family dinner to the highly contentious nuclear one, but they should be validated for these feelings. It's also important that children feel that some parts of their lives are continuing as before, so changing the food they eat, or the time of day when they eat it, might not be the best idea. Kids are trying to make sense of belonging to two families, so they may want to compare the dinners at each parent's house.

It's not just the children who must adjust to post-divorce dinners. For the parent, now single, it's an extra challenge to shop, cook, and clean up without the help of another adult. There may be more conflict introduced as a single parent turns to her children to help with some aspect of cooking or cleanup that the other parent did when they were still married.

With only one parent at the table, the conversation might feel less lively, or the small number of participants may make dinnertime feel too intense. One newly divorced mother of an eleven-year-old daughter felt that it was too much pressure to go from being a trio to a duo at dinner. She asked her daughter for ideas to make dinner more comfortable. Together they decided to bring something to read aloud—an article from the newspaper, an online blog, or a poem—that could bring in another voice to liven things up a little so that they weren't just staring at each other. Another family with several children designated one night a week as a night to invite friends and neighbors over, to give a feeling of abundance at a time when they felt such loss.

When a parent remarries

When a stepparent enters the scene, the bonds and loyalties among family members are reshuffled. The dinner table is a prime place to experience the sea change. As Dr. Patricia Papernow, a nationally renowned expert on stepfamilies explains: "Dinner is a time when children are reminded of how dramatically their family has changed. The new couple relationship is a long-awaited, wonderful gift to the adults. For kids, however, it often means a loss of parental attention and yet another in a series of difficult changes."[2] Kids now have to share a parent whose attention was exclusively theirs. If they start enjoying this new adult, they may feel disloyal to the parent who is no longer there. Meanwhile, the new couple may yearn for some time alone.

Papernow describes the disequilibrium further. The strongest and oldest bonds will be between the parent and children, as they share years of history and an implicit understanding of "how we do things in our family." This parent sits squarely on the inside of the family, closest to everyone—the stepparent, the kids, and even the ex-spouse. By sharp contrast, the stepparent, Papernow explains, is "late to the party" and can feel like an unwanted outsider. This contrast between insider and outsider can create a lot of tension. They may not understand inside jokes, get the references to treasured family stories, or like the food that's served. The children might not want to explain themselves so that the stepparent can join in. The children's parent will have the difficult task of trying to bridge these two constituencies.

Papernow offers advice that might seem antithetical to maintaining family dinners, but can eventually make them more possible. She recommends that in stepfamilies, family members "spend lots of time in one-to-one relationships" because "building relationships one dyad at a time is easier than expecting a stepparent to blend right into a preexisting family."[3] When it comes to dinners, different subsets of pairs can take turns making an appetizer or a dessert (adult stepcouple, two stepsiblings, stepparent and stepchild, parent and child). The adult couple could set a night to go out alone once a week. Becoming a stepfamily takes time (usually years), resourcefulness, and patience before the family reaches a new equilibrium.

When a parent is ill

When a parent is ill, particularly if that parent is the one who usually cooks, dinner will change dramatically. But maintaining a dinner ritual, even if it has to be radically altered, can provide stability and normalcy to both children and adults. There are many ways that families can handle the cooking when the main chef is sidelined by illness. Children can pick up the slack, but they may already be feeling burdened and depleted by having a sick parent. If the parents ask them to pitch in by first asking what they feel ready to do, it will work better. Perhaps a teenager would be willing to make one dinner a week for the family or, with a sibling, help make some soups and stews on the weekend.

Well-meaning friends and neighbors often offer to bring dinners after surgery, during chemotherapy, or when a parent is confined to bed. Dr. Paula Rauch, director of Massachusetts General Hospital's Parenting at a Challenging Time Program, recommends designating a "captain of kindness," to help organize the well-wishers. This person lets friends know about the family's food preferences—"please no more lasagnas" or "only vegetable soups and salads." The designated captain of kindness sends out instructions about the best time and place to deliver the food, so that the family knows when to expect dinner and doesn't have to entertain the person making the delivery.[4]

Figuring out some ways to keep having family dinners when a parent is sick is important because it gives a sense that the family is still able to nourish everyone. Keeping the routine going is key, even if it means having takeout food every night. Some families may want to agree that the dinner table is the one place that illness is excluded and decide not speak about it while they are having dinner together. Other families might prefer to let family members ask questions and raise worries at dinner—the one time of day when everyone is present.

CHANGING CONVERSATION, CHANGING THE FAMILY

Bruce and Martina were ready to divorce when they came for couples therapy as a last-ditch effort. Bruce was a stay-at-home father of their two teenagers, and Martina worked long hours as a software programmer. This arrangement suited Bruce much better than Martina. He had been laid off a decade earlier and found that he preferred taking care of the home front to working. Martina was able to support the family, but she often felt envious of her husband's greater intimacy with the children, and she worried that time was running out on getting to know them before they were out the door to college.

Dinner was a time when their parenting roles were particularly apparent. Bruce cooked and served dinner, and then liked to engage the kids in political debate about topics of the day. Martina, who had emigrated from Germany and spoke English as her third language, often felt left out.

"He can lecture them about events all over the world, and I just sit there," she explained. "I leave the table as soon as I finish eating."

I realized that Martina felt that she didn't have a place at the table; she was more of a guest than a parent. I asked her how she'd like dinner to be different. She took in a deep breath. "I want to know what the kids did during the day," she began. "I know Bruce has already heard all of that because he's been home with them for hours. I want to ask them how they feel about things that happened to them. Bruce is only interested in intellectual topics."

It was clear that she was just warming up. "I also want the kids to speak German at the table occasionally, and I want Bruce to cook German foods some of the time. They know so much more about his side of the family. And one more thing: When there's a disagreement with the kids, I want Bruce to take my side rather than ganging up on me."

Bruce had ideas as well. "I don't want Martina to introduce major rules at the table. You bark orders at them about their homework and how they have to get after-school jobs. It's just not relaxing for us."

"But dinner is the only time I have to try to influence what the kids do," Martina interjected.

Bruce gently suggested that she might catch more bees with honey. "If you enjoyed the kids, they'd be more likely to listen to you when you told them to do something."

Martina bristled at this. "I don't need to be told how to be a mother," she said.

Keeping in mind that dinner is a stage upon which many of their dynamics unfold, I thought that improvising a few new interactions could be helpful. Mindful that there were many problematic exchanges, I didn't want to overwhelm them with too much homework. I suggested two experiments, one for each to try. Turning to Martina, I said, "What if you try to jump into a conversation that Bruce had begun?" And to Bruce I said, "What if you start the meal by asking Martina about her day, and include some questions about her feelings? Then Martina might feel there was room for her to ask similar questions of the children."

The following week, the couple reported that dinners had lasted longer. Bruce observed that the kids were more relaxed and that the rest of the night went more smoothly. Martina added that they actually had fun.

This was just a start, but it was a success they could build on.

FOOD METAPHORS IN SEX THERAPY

Don't get me wrong. I'm not suggesting that you work on your sexual relationship at the family dinner table. Nor am I advocating for the aphrodisiacal powers of oysters, chocolate, or avocados. I'm going in a different direction as I close out this chapter, because I'm a big fan of using food metaphors in therapy. Since food is a language that everyone speaks—and because it easily taps into topics such as desire, appetite, asking for what you want, and trying new things—it's ripe for riffing on in therapy.

Food metaphors are particularly apt when talking about sex, which is, after all, a type of appetite. The most common sexual problem that couples seek help for from a therapist is loss of sexual desire—a partner's loss of appetite for the other. It turns out that the things that can reawaken a person's taste for food are pretty similar to what you might do to regain a hearty sexual appetite.

For starters, there is a famous French saying *l'appetit vient en mangeant,* or in English it's "the appetite is in the eating." In other words, even if you're not that hungry when you sit down to eat, if the food is good, you might discover that you're hungrier than you thought. Similarly, if couples engage in sex only when they are feeling desirous, or hungry for sex, this will limit the occasions for sexual encounters. Instead, they can ask each other, "What makes for an inviting and appetizing sexual encounter?" Perhaps, it's a candlelit bedroom, a chance to take a nap, or a backrub. "What can I do to get you to the bedroom so that you are willing to partake of what I can offer you?"

For many couples, particularly those who have been married a long time, desire will follow, not precede, the start of a sexual encounter. Sex researchers have discovered, for example, that many women who have been married ten years or more report experiencing desire only *after* foreplay and arousal have begun.[5] This scientific discovery flies in the face of years of the presumed sequence of sexual activity, i.e., desire preceding arousal. It has led sex researchers to ask women, "Are you receptive to having sex?" rather than, "Do you desire sex?" This receptivity to sex seems similar to a person being willing to try a new food, even if they didn't come to the table ravenous.

Food metaphors can also help frame conversations about what a person prefers and the notion that tastes can change without the meal being considered a failure. What feels satisfying? What do I want, and what do you want? Do you want to try something new, or go back to the same trusty dish? These are all questions that work in talking both about food and about sex. They're questions that help ease couples into talking about sex, since, by comparison, we are so much more practiced in talking about food.

Talking about food, reconfiguring cooking roles, and experimenting with dinner table conversation are all ways that I think about family dinners as a therapist. I've come to see the kitchen as an annex to my therapy office, and often a much more important place for new behaviors to get started and take root. Family dinners can be recipes for therapeutic growth as well as the best part of the day.

10

Extending the Dinner Table
to the Wide World

Dinner sits at the hub of a wheel with spokes extending in many directions. One spoke is an opportunity to have a conversation about economic disparities that lead to poverty, diabetes, and obesity; another spoke reminds us to protect the environment by not wasting food and by eating in a "green way"; while other spokes serve as starting points for school-age kids to become activists or as bridges to fund-raisers in the service of social justice. Dinner can also be a passport to other countries. Food is the ultimate connector—to our environment, to our fellow citizens who don't have enough to eat, and to our basic humanity—because everyone must eat to live. This chapter is about some of the ways that the dinner table can be a classroom for global citizenship and a jumping off point for making a difference in the world.

EXPAND THE GUEST LIST: DINNER AS A PASSPORT

A couple of times a year my dinner table becomes an international hub. If you closed your eyes, you might think you were at the Olympics dining hall, with young adults from countries as far flung as China, Pakistan, India, Italy, Ecuador, Greece, and Saudi Arabia. These gatherings happen because my husband, a Boston University professor, teaches a weekly journalism class to about a dozen international graduate students. The class is aimed at improving their writing skills and helping them learn the folkways of living and working in the United States—everything from the rules of baseball to the most common swearwords, to the American teaching practice of asking open-ended questions in class. The class also serves as a soft landing place for homesick young adults who, often for the first time in their lives, are living far away from their families. The students form tight bonds with one another, and they know that they have an adult, my husband, to call on in an emergency—a trip to the ER, a bout of insomnia after covering the Marathon bombings, or shock after a fellow student's fatal bicycle accident.

Every September, we invite these students to our home for dinner. What began as our welcome-to-America-dinner has become much more—it's now an opportunity for us to learn about different countries and cultures. Along the way, we've been inspired by the courage it takes to travel halfway around the world to get an advanced degree in a field of communication when English is neither your first nor even your second language.

A week before the dinner party, we send a note to all the students asking about food preferences and allergies. Usually they reply that they eat everything, with a few adding that they are vegetarians or observe Halal. Food allergies seem distinctly American, or maybe these students are too polite to make special requests. (When I invite my students, a group of psychiatry residents, for dinner, a list of verboten foods almost always comes back: No mushrooms, no tree nuts, no lactose, no carbs, and "nothing with a mother.")

For the first few years, the international journalism dinner was a potluck. We made it that way because we believed that the students would like to share their home country cuisine. But few actually had the time or the inclination to cook, so after a few dinners that featured takeout Styrofoam tubs, we realized that what these students craved was a home-cooked meal, even if the food was strange and unfamiliar. So, my husband, ever the teacher, decided to create an early Thanksgiving celebration where he could teach them about different holiday foods and their meanings. But turkeys are hard to find in September. The butcher offered to sell us turkey wings, breasts, and drumsticks, which we could have assembled like a Lego sculpture. Luckily, we tracked down a whole one at a poultry farm. Also on the menu was our family's time-honored Thanksgiving lineup: sweet potato pudding with marshmallows, stuffing, roasted vegetables, cranberry sauce, and pecan and apple pies.

Teaching about culture, of course, goes both ways. Dinner was called for 7 p.m., but at 6:45, Ahmed, a young man from Saudi Arabia, arrived, explaining that it is considered polite in his country to arrive early. At 7:30, Primm from Thailand arrived, explaining that it's considered polite to be 30 minutes late. Almost no one came empty-handed, bringing tea and silk pajamas from China, a wall hanging from Pakistan, flowers, wine, and scarves. This graciousness is lovely and unexpected. I now always pack some gifts when I travel to another country in case I'm invited to someone's home.

The students were homesick for their families, and even though the food was strange, my husband and I, roughly the ages of their parents, functioned *in locus parentis* for the evening. Over dinner we talked about many topics: the ways that their fellow American students interacted with them; the foods they ate when they were sick and the ones they just found comforting; the differences in marriage laws in their countries; the media they read every day; and how often they were in touch with their families.

After many of these dinners, I'm still intrigued by the ways food practices are both similar and startlingly different. In particular, I've looked

HOW TO BRING NEW CULTURAL EXPERIENCES TO YOUR DINNER TABLE

- Contact the principal at your children's school to find out if there are new students arriving from abroad who might enjoy having dinner with your family.
- Contact a local church or synagogue, as many religious organizations have programs to welcome families arriving from other countries.
- If you attended a college in the area where you now live, contact the alumni affairs office. Inquire about whether there are programs for hosting students from other countries who are currently attending your alma mater.
- Seek out food festivals in your area.

CONVERSATION STARTERS WHEN YOU'RE HOSTING INTERNATIONAL GUESTS

- What foods do you eat when you need some comfort?
- What foods do you eat when you're sick with a cold, a fever, or a stomachache?
- When do you have your main meal at home?
- What are the most significant holidays in your country and in your family? Are there special foods you eat as part of a celebration?
- What is your favorite home-cooked meal?
- Who comes to a special family dinner in your home? Who do you consider to be your family?
- What is the meaning of food in your family?
- Are there are any roles around shopping, preparation, serving, cleaning up that are defined by gender?
- Are there any foods you would never eat? Many cultures have a fermented delicacy that most members of that culture revere but people outside the culture might find repulsive, such as shark corpse left to decompose for several months (Greenland); *Chicha,* a blend of boiled maize and human saliva (Ecuador); maggot cheese, swarming with live insect larvae (Sardinia); *kimchi,* rotten cabbage (Korea); 100-year-old eggs (China). People from other cultures sometimes turn up their noses at our blue cheese, declaring that it smells like unwashed T-shirts.
- Are there any foods you've eaten here that you thought you wouldn't like but did? Any foods you found unpleasant?

into the different foods that people eat when they aren't feeling well or when they need a helping of comfort.

LEARN ABOUT OTHER CULTURES THROUGH EXPLORING "INVALID" FOODS

Over the years I have become intrigued by the cultural differences and similarities that show up around the foods that children eat when they are feeling poorly. Sejal, from India, told me that when she was sick as a child she ate rice flour blended with a grinder, cooked in water, and then mixed with yogurt into a porridge consistency. Khyati, another Indian student, ate *khichdi*—a mixture of rice and mung dai, a form of green lentils pressure-cooked with a little bit of salt and turmeric. This was then paired with buttermilk and the end result was a pale yellow. A Chinese journalist remembered that she ate *jook*—a soup made with chicken stock and a piece of ginger root, boiled with rice until the rice is broken down and the soup is the consistency of a watery porridge. Aspasia, a journalist from Greece, ate angel hair pasta soup, accompanied by small pieces of boiled chicken, with a lot of lemon juice. Bibi, a student from Kuwait, ate plain chicken broth with small pieces of chicken. So many of these "invalid foods" are carbohydrates, the building blocks for serotonin; these are the foods that people with atypical depression often crave. Maybe sushi, porridge, noodle soup, and angel pasta soup are invalid foods because of their common carbohydrate base.

Many of these foods are yellow or white. I've heard that yellow is a cue to eat and that a lot of yellow foods—such as bananas, corn, lemons, and squash—are brimming with Vitamin C, which is good for the immune system. Perhaps there's an evolutionary reason to eat yellow foods when we are sick.

A lot of "sick" foods include the generous use of spices, particularly when someone has a cold or fever. One young man from Nigeria told me that when he had a bad cold his mother made him a pepper soup—a super spicy brown broth loaded with chicken, veggies, and plantain. Capsaicin, a natural compound in peppers, can help thin mucous and clear stuffy noses. Salt, which flavors chicken soup, also helps to thin mucous. A young man from Jordan remembered eating lots of onions, fresh mint, and radishes, along with a drink made with fresh ginger, lemon, and honey.

According to evolutionary biologists Jennifer Billing and Paul Sherman, who looked at almost 100 cookbooks from thirty-six countries, certain spices serve an antibacterial function.[1] Garlic, onion, allspice, and oregano inhibit every bacterium they have been tested on. And some foods are more powerful when paired with others. For example, lemon juice and lime juice act synergistically to enhance the antibacterial effects of certain spices. And such spices as garlic, ginger, cinnamon, and chilies have for centuries been used to attack pneumonia, high blood pressure, and nausea.

What do you want when you're sick? Do you gravitate toward the foods your parents gave you when you had a fever or a cold? Or do you find yourself craving a food that has nothing to do with your cultural background but that may have universal medicinal properties, such as chicken soup?

When I think of my older son's food preferences when he was sick, I'm hard-pressed to find either a cultural explanation or a medicinal one. He'd raise his head wanly off the couch pillow and ask for sushi and a vanilla milkshake. In retrospect, I think he was asking for comfort foods, not "sick foods." He was probably taking a mental health day rather than a sick day off from school.

MAKE CONNECTIONS TO FOOD JUSTICE

When I was a girl, my mother would admonish me if I didn't finish everything on my plate: "Children are starving in Biafra. You should be grateful for your food and eat it all." This was my first inkling of the way that my dinner could connect beyond my own plate. But, there are really dozens of leaps to make from a dinner plate to social justice issues.

For starters, take environmentalism: The carbon footprint of a family dinner expands when the food is transported from far away, so eating locally grown foods is one way to help the environment. Food that's thrown away will end up in landfills, decomposing and giving off methane, a greenhouse gas twenty-five times more powerful in global warming than carbon dioxide. So avoiding food waste is helpful to our planet. A family of four is estimated to waste the equivalent of more than $2,000 a year on food that gets thrown out. Think how far that money could go toward feeding the more than one in six children in America that are hungry.[2]

Income disparities and injustices are also magnified by food choices: fast-food restaurants that produce supersize portions of high-fat, salty, and sugary foods are prevalent in low-income neighborhoods, where there are also more liquor stores and mini-marts than grocery stores selling fresh produce.[3] Racial disparities also play a role in who has access to healthy food: Compared to white households, there are four times as many black and Hispanic households that are considered "food insecure."[4]

Tristram Stuart, an international authority on food waste, runs the global organization Feedback. Feedback is aimed at raising awareness and offering solutions to the problem of food waste in affluent countries.[5] Tristram is a "freegan"—he takes food from bins outside supermarkets and gleans perfectly good (though cosmetically imperfect) produce from farms and redistributes it. Most notably, he uses this scavenged food in his Feeding 5000 campaign, where 5,000 people eat for free in big outdoor festivals, consuming food that would otherwise have gone to waste.

I spoke to Tristram by phone from his office in London to find out how he thinks children and families can help tackle the problem of food waste.

"I have tried to reawaken the proximity that families have to their food," he said. "Supermarkets give the illusion of a cornucopia, of infinite produce. It's hard in that environment, when you see stacks of bananas, to connect to a plantation in Ecuador, to all the bananas that were thrown out because they didn't look so perfect, to the deforestation that went into growing those bananas. My efforts are to reconnect people to how they treat their food."[6]

He explained that once families understand these connections, they'll intuitively figure out ways to save food scraps, use leftovers, and make smoothies out of brown bananas. He added that children are the ambassadors of this movement who can be counted on to nag their parents to be better global citizens. Children are quick studies. They "get" how silly and shameful it is to throw out perfectly good food just because it's discolored or misshapen.

Talking to your children about these connections is one way to get them thinking about becoming food justice activists. But there are other ways that are more action-oriented.

Cultivate a gardening activist

The garden can be a place to grow beans and to cultivate activism. Roger Doiron, who spearheaded the Obama White House garden by mobilizing a network of gardening activists across the country, describes gardening as a subversive activity.

"Food is a form of power, and by growing your own food, then you're taking power away from those who have power over your health."[7] He also asserts that gardening is a healthy gateway drug to other forms of food freedom: Once you start growing your own food, you have to learn to cook and preserve it.

At the Ford School in Lynn, Massachusetts, just a few miles north of Boston, there's a garden built over blacktop. There you will find elementary school activist gardeners planting taro, jalapeño peppers, and more than thirty other vegetables, alongside a veteran activist, David Gass. David heads up the neighborhood advocacy group, Highlands Coalition, but his activist roots go back to 1964 and the tumultuous days of voter registration in Mississippi. The elementary school is home to families who have emigrated from countries as widespread as El Salvador, Haiti, Ethiopia, Iraq, Cambodia, and the Dominican Republic, and where 90 percent of kids qualify for free breakfasts.

In 2008, the principal, Dr. Claire Crane, spearheaded the creation of this 1,500-square-foot garden, which hugs a brick wall running the length of the school. The goal was simple, but bold: to engage the students in healthy eating, given that their obesity rates were twice as high as the national average.[8]

The genius of the garden is the way that the surrounding families have gotten involved. Many of the neighbors bring sophisticated agricultural knowledge from their home countries, where they grew up on farms before immigrating to Lynn, a poor city and a veritable food desert. Sometimes this knowledge brings surprises: A Nigerian man harvested what Gass thought was a weed. It turned out to be a leafy green, callaloo, that he cooked up for lunch. Another neighbor pulled up another "weed," which was really a Cambodian herb that jazzed up some chicken soup.

The garden has transformed the neighborhood, which used to be plagued by gang activity. Since the creation of this garden and another one down the street, there has been a dramatic decrease in drugs and shootings. Gass told me about a family that wanted to move out of the neighborhood because of the prevalence of crime. Grateful for the increased sense of safety, this family now contributes rainwater into the garden from the roof of their house.

Gass, who has worked in housing development and real estate, understands the ins and outs of banks and evictions, a knowledge that came in handy with a three-generation Cambodian family that was about to be evicted. Gass advocated for them at the local bank and prevented their eviction. The family, which had farmed for the Khmer Rouge before moving to Lynn, asked what it could do in return. Gass asked the family members for their help in the garden: The family made trellises and planted long beans, ginseng, and bok choy—contributions that were novel delicacies to many kids at the school.

"Kids who don't eat vegetables light up when they eat those long beans," Gass told me.

When I go to the Ford School to help run community dinners, I love to stroll through the garden, a messy, packed area where low-tech materials make high-tech solutions. Most crops are planted in raised soil beds, but tomato plants are growing in five-gallon buckets, and chives are sprouting from a plastic shoe organizer that hangs off a fence. Raised beds are watered by drip irrigation; there are no pesticides used on the fifty-plus different species growing on a block-long narrow space. There's also an aquaponics project: A large fish tank supports the growth of plants, which are nourished by goldfish excrement. There's vertical gardening too, with pipes— recycled from a generous plumbing company—that stretch six feet into the air. And there's a worm factory churning through food scraps, producing top-grade compost to nourish the soil for the future. The children at the Ford Elementary School help with the planting and harvesting, and they are the proud winners of several prizes at the annual Topsfield Fair, America's oldest agricultural fair.

In the process, they're encouraged to teach their families what they've learned about healthy eating. The hands-on engagement gets kids to form a strong connection to fresh, healthy food. Wandering through the garden, I notice some laminated signs sticking out of the ground. From Michael Pollan's *Food Rules*: "Eat food. Not too much. Mostly plants." Another sign reads: "Avoid food with ingredients that a third-grader can't pronounce." And a third: "Try new kinds of plants, animals, and fungi, not just new foods. More diversity in species is nutritionally better." The hope is that this knowledge of healthy food will help drive down the skyrocketing obesity rates in this community.

The children at the Ford School are part of a growing movement of "Farm to School" programs that improve the health of children and communities with such activities as planting school gardens, teaching cooking, bringing local foods to school cafeterias, and taking farm field trips. Across the country, schools are becoming champions of improving food access and health to their students. As of 2013, Farm to School programs have reached more than 38,000 schools and 21 million children in all 50 states.[9]

Alice Waters—the founder of the celebrated Berkeley, California, restaurant Chez Panisse and the Edible Schoolyard, a national project to bring gardens to public schools—calls for a revolution in public education, which she named the "Delicious Revolution." This revolution will occur "when the hearts and minds of our children are captured by a school lunch curriculum, enriched with experience in the garden, and sustainability will become the lens through which they see the world."[10] The children who garden at the Ford School are on the front lines of the Delicious Revolution.

If you want your children to be part of the Delicious Revolution, you can plant gardens in your backyard (or in your front yard, if that's where the sun shines), or in pots that perch on windowsills. Gardening, at school or at home, instills a deep appreciation for food and for the people who grew it. There's nothing quite as powerful as growing your own fruit from seed and then eating it if you want to develop a respect for food and the work that goes into creating it. This appreciation can be the first step toward advocating for access to safe, healthy food and for protection of our valuable resources. When children are involved in planting, watering, staking, fertilizing, and harvesting a cup of raspberries, they'll think twice about squandering a single berry. When children appreciate the work that goes into growing their food, they learn to become stewards of the land.

Engage your kids in saving the planet

I was shocked to learn that 40 percent of food produced in the United States never gets eaten. It's tossed away on over-portioned plates at home; it rots

TIPS FOR CULTIVATING CHILD GARDENERS

- Let your children choose what to plant, making sure that some of their choices are trusty winners.
- Encourage digging, as holes in the ground are interesting places to spot worms and to muck around in.
- Use spray guns, hoses, sprinklers, and buckets to water your garden. These waterworks will all get the job done, while amusing your children.
- Enjoy your harvest. It's the big payoff. If you have a bounty, you can make a preserve to save for the winter, or to give away, proudly, as a gift from your garden. You can also donate extra vegetables to a local soup kitchen or food pantry.
- Start seedlings indoors in egg cartons, milk containers, and juice cans. Seeds will sprout and then shoot up fairly quickly, enough to capture a young child's attention.
- Keep an eye out for insects that you may unearth. Don't assume that they're all pests. Look them up first, and find out what good or ill they are doing. The garden is a morality play in action.
- Build a scarecrow to keep birds from eating your garden. Build a simple frame with tree branches and then dress it with old clothes. Make a head out of papier-mâché, or stuff a woolen hat with straw and attach cut-up straws or other plastic pieces to make a face. Hang pie tins or other noisemakers from the arms.
- Make teepees with five or more poles tied together at the top. Plant below with pole beans, cucumbers, miniature pumpkins, or gourds.
- Use bendable twigs, such as crabapple, willow, or dogwood, to make sculptures and structures such as arches, figures, and nests. To make arches, plant two vertical sticks into the ground and weave twigs between them.
- Grow fragrant flowers like roses, lilacs, peonies, and honeysuckle. Decades from now, your kids will be transported back to their childhood gardens on the scent of these flowers.
- Plant a strawberry or a raspberry patch. These provide hours of entertainment, as children have to hunt for the fruit, much as they would if

they were looking for hidden treasures or Easter eggs. Also, new berries keep showing up over many weeks or months.

- Grow vegetables that come in surprising colors, including candy-striped beets, yellow carrots, and purple potatoes.
- Plant flowers that will attract butterflies such as milkweed, bee balm, thistle, and parsley.
- Plant edible flowers like pansies, Johnny-jump-ups, dandelions, nasturtiums, and violets. There is something magical about eating a salad or a soup that is dotted with flowers from your garden.
- Be sure to have your soil tested before you start planting. You can do it yourself with a soil-test kit, or you can hire a testing lab. Make sure that the previous home dwellers haven't left behind lead and that the pH of the soil is as close to neutral as possible.

in refrigerators when we buy too much; it gets thrown out by supermarkets when nonregulated expiration dates dictate that perfectly good food is over the hill; and it is disposed of on farms that throw away imperfectly sized and shaped fruits and vegetables.

It's estimated that American families will throw out the equivalent of $165 billion worth of food each year.[11] The environmental cost of this waste begins with the toxic gas methane that is given off when food scraps decompose in landfills. This accounts for 25 percent of all methane emissions.[12] If food waste were a country, it would rank third in greenhouse gas emissions after China and the United States.[13]

When one in six Americans lacks a secure supply of food, and billions more lack food globally, wasting perfectly good food also becomes a moral issue. If waste was cut by even 15 percent, the food saved could feed more than 25 millions Americans every year.[14] Pope Francis recently lent his voice to this issue on World Environment Day when he said, "Throwing away food is like stealing from the table of those who are poor and hungry."[15]

Many organizations have sprung up to redistribute excess food from restaurants, college cafeterias, and supermarkets and bring it to shelters and soup kitchens. There are also efforts to glean surplus produce from farms and transport it to those in need.[16] Some states, like California, Arizona, Oregon, and Colorado, have passed bills allowing growers to receive a tax credit when they give excess produce to food banks. Certain corporations are beginning to alter their production practices to cut down on wasted food. There is much to be done.

Every day, families that think globally and act locally can also make a difference in cutting down on food waste.

Prevent unnecessary food waste with better **refrigerator** and **freezer** practices:

- Don't let ice build up in your freezer; this cuts down on space for keeping food (and uses up extra energy).
- Store yogurt or cheese (foods with a low safety risk) on upper fridge shelves, which are slightly warmer.
- Store meat, poultry, and fish (foods with a high safety risk) on the lower shelves, which are cooler.
- Put fruits and vegetables that have a tendency to rot or break down— peppers, mushrooms, berries, and pears—in a low-humidity drawer in the fridge.
- To conserve energy, don't leave the fridge open, even when you're doing a quick activity like pouring milk in your cereal.
- Put condiments on the fridge door, as this is the warmest part.
- Keep your fridge at 40 degrees or below, as bacteria grow most rapidly between 40 and 140 degrees.
- Freeze unused ingredients rather than waiting for them to rot. You can freeze foods before the "use by" date and then defrost them when you need them, and use within twenty-four hours. You can freeze eggs, meat, and bread, for example, when they are close to their expiration date

Prevent unnecessary food waste with better **buying, preparation,** and **serving** practices:

- The size of the average American plate expanded by 36 percent from 1960 to 2007. Switching to eating off a smaller plate can help prevent waste.

- Read and critically assess the expiration labels on food. The "sell by," "use by," and "best before" dates do not usually pertain to the safety of the food and are not regulated by any government agency. Instead, the dating system misleads you into thinking that you must discard food that actually may still be perfectly fine. As a result, we needlessly throw out billions of pounds of food.[17]

- Buy imperfect products, like misshapen vegetables.

- If you find that you have bought too much food, or if you are going to be away and your food will rot in your absence, you can donate this perfectly good food to a food bank or homeless shelter. Consult the Feeding America Food Bank Locator to find an organization near you.

- Create interesting meals from leftovers: My favorite recycled recipe is tomato bread soup, which is a delicious way to use up stale bread and ends of loaves and imperfect tomatoes (see recipe that follows).

- Or repurpose food items: You can use leftover tea to marinate meat before cooking. Or reuse an old tea bag to make a cold brew and then use it as a cleaning solution to remove grease and grime on mirrors.[18]

TOMATO BREAD SOUP

2 tablespoons olive oil

1 onion, diced

1 celery stalk, diced

1 carrot stick, diced

2 cloves garlic, minced

1 fennel bulb, diced

2 cups stale bread, cut into cubes (if you only have fresh bread, you can lightly toast it)

1 (28-ounce) can plum tomatoes (pureed in a food processor) or 4 fresh tomatoes

1 quart vegetable or chicken stock

¼ cup red wine

½ cup chopped fresh basil leaves

Grated Parmesan cheese

In a Dutch oven or heavy soup pan, heat the oil and throw in the onion, celery, carrots, garlic, and fennel, sautéing over medium heat until soft. Then toss in the bread and stir for about 1 minute, or until it is coated in oil.

Add the tomatoes, basil leaves, stock, and wine, and simmer over low heat for about 30 minutes. Season with salt and pepper.

Serve with generous amounts of Parmesan cheese on top.

TEACH KIDS TO COMPOST:
TURN WASTE INTO GOLD

Composting is a cheap, natural way to get something from nothing; in a few months your discarded garbage is transformed into a nutrient-rich food for your garden. Composting at home for a year can save global-warming gasses equivalent to what your washing machine produces in three months.[19]

Composting is an easy job to assign to a child because it's basically just dumping food scraps into a pile, where they will rot and turn into wonderful fertilizer while reducing your flow of garbage. To begin, you can make or purchase a plastic or wooden bin (often subsidized by your local government because it wants to divert materials from its waste stream). If grass clippings and shredded leaves are available toss them together in alternating layers. Otherwise, just get started with whatever food scraps you have on hand—eggshells, tea bags, coffee grinds, potato peels, discarded pumpkins, watermelon rinds, tough broccoli stalks, and almost anything else. Best to leave out fish bones or meat since those could attract a party of skunks and rodents making whoopee in your backyard.

The compost pile also needs oxygen and water. Use a shovel or a pitchfork to lift everything and turn it around, aerating the mess, and bringing different materials into contact with one another (which helps the rotting process). Do this at least once a month, or whenever you think of it. Water the pile or collect rainwater and use that to keep it moist but not soggy.

If you really want to go all-in, buy bags full of compost starters—bugs and worms—but your own worms will eventually make their way to your compost, where they'll eat it and excrete the aftereffects.

How long it will take the composting process to transform your garbage into rich fertilizer is a bit of a mystery, but you'll know it's ready to spread on vegetable and flowerbeds when the stuff at the bottom of the bin is textured, blacker than regular soil, and when you can't recognize the disparate parts.

EAT LOCAL, EAT GREEN

A typical American meal contains ingredients from five foreign countries. After all, we've become a culture that wants the food it wants, any time of year. For instance, we eat apples in the spring from New Zealand, watermelon in the winter from Chile, and asparagus in the fall from Argentina. Even domestically grown produce travels an average of 1,500 miles before it's sold.[20] All that globetrotting on the part of our food dramatically increases fuel consumption and pollution. So eating locally grown foods is a tangible way to make the environment cleaner. Can you eat one dinner a week with foods that are grown within 100 miles of where you live? It's easy enough to do in the summer when farmer's markets are overflowing with produce, but what can you rustle up in January? In Massachusetts, I can make meal of roasted potatoes, beets, parsnips, and apples with a locally caught cod, or a frittata with onions, herbs grown on the windowsill, and spinach. (Make sure the spinach is sold loose rather than in a plastic container to keep down the fossil fuels expended in production.) You might think you could throw in some frozen asparagus for this experiment, but frozen vegetables triple the carbon footprint.[21] Eating locally grown foods is not an easy challenge, unless you devote your life to it, as some do. I know I couldn't go without coffee for more than a day.

EAT LOWER ON THE FOOD CHAIN

The Natural Resources Defense Council estimates that if Americans eliminated as little as a one-quarter pound serving of beef per week, the reduction in global warming gas emission would be the equivalent of taking four to six million cars off the road.[22] That's because beef production, more than the production of pork, chicken, fruits, or vegetables, takes the greatest toll on the environment. Cows release methane gas in their manure. Cows also require wide expanses of grazing land, usually the result of deforestation. And then there is all the irrigation needed to pump the water needed to grow the corn to feed the cows. Besides, eating less meat and more fruits and vegetables has the added bonus of being less expensive and better for your health.

COOK TO RAISE MONEY

Some people raise money and awareness for a charity by biking, walking, or running, but you can also cook or bake your way to making a difference. When my mother died after a long struggle with cancer, I wanted to do something that could help stop this disease from claiming more lives. When I thought of all the bake sales I had participated in at my sons' schools, it occurred to me that cooking was more my speed than soliciting pledges for a walk-a-thon. My teenage sons were also reeling from their grandmother's death. I thought they would appreciate the opportunity to raise money for cancer research, and I knew I'd enjoy talking about my mother while hanging out together in the kitchen.

I asked them if they'd like to make portable dinner parties. The idea was simple: People could buy a dinner from us, we could cook and deliver it, and the proceeds would go to the Dana-Farber Cancer Institute in Boston. And so we began "Serving up a Cure"—or dinner parties to go. My sons wrote emails soliciting their friends' parents, designed a menu, and purchased restaurant-size aluminum containers for transport. Then they called up their friends and enlisted them to help. Before I knew it, the kitchen was chock-a-block with teenagers chopping, cutting, and assembling dinners into a box.

My sons also wrote the menu, parodying the over-the-top menu prose of trendy restaurants, and promising slightly more than we were going to deliver. It featured:

- Mediterranean Flatbread—"Flatbread topped with a mix of caramelized onions, chiffonade of kale, thyme, asiago, and olive nicoise."

- Roman-Style Artichokes—"A ready-to-eat artichoke heart steamed and rubbed in mint, parsley, and olive oil, served in its own juices."
- Rice Salad—"A refreshing mix of rustic wild rices with craisins and Alabama pecans finished with mint and orange zest."
- Chicken Roulades—"A tenderized chicken breast rolled to perfection with fresh garden pesto, and a stuffing made from toasted pine nuts, roasted garlic, mozzarella, and kalamata olives."
- Dessert was homemade vanilla ice cream served with homemade chocolate-dipped biscotti, accompanied by balsamic-macerated berries.

Not too shabby!

We made dozens of these dinners and charged $50 a person, raising thousands of dollars in the process, and having a blast. I think my children learned about the deep satisfaction that comes from contributing to something bigger than them. Together, we had the experience of doing good in the world while having a good time.

CHANGING THE WORLD ONE LOAF AT A TIME

Challah for Hunger (CfH) is a national organization that "bakes for a difference." The organization leverages the same idea I had with my sons—having fun in the kitchen while doing good in the world—across sixty college campuses. Founded in 2004 by Eli Winkelman, a Scripps College student, the idea was to bake challahs (braided Jewish loaves of bread), sell them, and send the money to support Muslim refugees in Sudan.

As Bill Clinton described the organization—"Jewish girls baking Jewish bread saving Muslim kids' lives in Africa that have been overlooked by other people."[23] But actually, it's not just Jewish girls. The organization attracts Muslim, Buddhist, Christian, and atheist male and female students. Carly Zimmerman, the current director of CfH, explained: " We are rooted in Jewish values, but gathering around food and wanting to make a difference attracts all kinds of students."[24]

Over the past 10 years, the organization has raised about $600,000. Half of that money goes to fight genocide in Darfur. The other half goes to local social justice organizations selected by each individual chapter. Caryn Roth, an adviser to college chapters, explained that it's not the bread that gets sent to Darfur. Instead, the profits from selling the bread might pay for a solar cooker for Sudanese women who previously risked being raped when they had to leave their camp to look for wood. With the money from the sale of only six challah loaves, these women can now afford a slow cooker with two pots per family. Making this connection between baking and activism might be the greatest thing since sliced bread for many busy college students wanting to make a difference in the world.

The MIT chapter of CfH meets most Thursday nights for six hours of mixing, kneading, and baking. On a frigid February night I joined this group of about 10 future astrophysicists, neuroscientists, and engineers. As they compared problem sets due for the next day's classes, I thought, "Baking isn't rocket science, but I'm baking with rocket scientists!"

These college students come to bake for a variety of reasons. One young woman was directing a play above the kitchen, and the yeasty smell of baking bread drew her downstairs. Caroline, a talkative woman who grew up doing a lot of charity work through her church, told me she came because she liked the bread and stayed because it was awesome. Still others, like Jill, the head of this club, are like family members who come to the dinner table for the food but linger because of the conversation. The baking brings them to the club, but talk about social justice keeps them coming back.

By 11 p.m., the seventy-five loaves were done. As was customary for this group, they made three kinds of challah—plain, cinnamon with sugar, and Nutella. Plus, there is always one special flavor of the week. That week it was Reese's Cup challah. Other weeks they've made challah with peanut butter and jelly, pumpkin pie filling, and "challa-ween" (candy challah). One student tells me confidentially that while all the challahs are vegan, they advertise them as "plain" or "vegan," since some students don't like the sound of "vegan challah." Then they delivered them hot out of the oven to dorms all over campus. For a few minutes, the club members were campus rock stars, as their fellow students were so grateful to have their Thursday night problem sets interrupted by a bread delivery. There will be no trace of the bread by Friday.

This group sends half its weekly profits (about $300) to Darfur, and the other half to a local organization, Food for Free, which rescues fresh food that would otherwise go to waste and distributes it within the local emergency food system. Five hours of work earns each baking participant a loaf of bread. That seems like ample payment, given the other perks and pleasures of the evening, such as one young man entertaining the group by juggling several dough balls. Over and over, this group of intense young scientists and engineers tell me how therapeutic it is to knead and punch the dough, what a stress reliever it is to bake bread. For an evening, they are separated from their phones and computer screens, since they would ruin their devices with their sticky, doughy fingers.

Advice from Challah for Hunger activists to other budding activists:

- Record everything when you start a project. Be organized and keep as much information as possible.
- Just "do it." Buy the ingredients, and gather friends together to bake.
- "Make for yourself a teacher," or find people you can learn from and then go learn from them.
- Start with the question "Why am I doing this?" and try to inspire others to ask the question.
- Collaborate with other organizations.
- Don't give up, even when there are obstacles like safety issues with food. Instead, get advice from someone in the food industry.
- Keep reminding yourself and the people you're working with about why the cause is important. Keep connecting back to the reason you are doing the cooking or the baking.

CHALLAH FOR HUNGER BREAD
(MAKES 2 FAMILY-SIZE LOAVES OR 6 INDIVIDUAL LOAVES)

The following recipe uses *instant* yeast. If you are using active dry or another kind of yeast you'll need to make modifications.

¾ cup sugar
½ cup vegetable oil
½ tablespoon salt
2½ cups water

6 to 8 cups all-purpose flour, divided

1 tablespoon instant yeast

Additional oil

Prep your space! Clean surfaces, hands, put hair up, and take off rings, etc.

Mix the sugar, ½ cup oil, salt, and water in a large bowl, mixing until everything is dissolved.

Add 3 cups of the flour and mix. You will not necessarily be able to get rid of all the clumps of flour yet; that's okay. Just keep going.

In a separate, small bowl, combine 1 tablespoon instant yeast with 1 cup of the flour. After the yeast has been thoroughly mixed into the flour, add the mixture to the dough bowl.

Continue adding flour, between 2 and 4 more cups. As your mixture becomes more solid, add the flour more and more slowly. Add flour until you reach the point when, if you press the dough *gently* with *clean* fingers, no dough sticks to your hands.

Let the dough rest for 10 minutes. Take a break! Then knead, using the heel of your hand, (not your fingers) for 6 minutes. (You may have to add some flour while kneading, but be conservative.)

Put the dough back in the bowl, cover with a skim of oil, and then drape a towel over the bowl; let it rise for at least 1 hour (but monitor it to make sure it doesn't overflow the bowl). You can let the dough rise overnight in the fridge (the rising process slows down in cooler temperatures).

Braid the dough and, if desired, add an egg wash. If you have time, let the loaf rise before you bake it. Bake at 350 degrees for 30 to 40 minutes, or until golden brown.

My note: If you are adding other ingredients (like garlic and herb, banana chunks, chocolate chips, or apple pie filler), the group uses the strand method. Once the dough is made, each pre-measured pound of dough is divided in half, and rolled out into an 8-inch snake. Make a trough down the middle of this strand, and sprinkle or spread on the toppings. Then pinch the strand back together and braid it. Then bring the strands together into a round shape.

Questions or comments? Contact Carly at carly@challahforhunger.org.

A PLOT OF LAND, A PLOT OF TIME

Dinner can be the secure base from which children explore the wider world. Food lies at the center of a living web that connects us as global citizens since we all have to eat to live. As stewards of the planet we need to share the limited and precious natural resources to grow our food. At dinner we can talk about these connections, and talk can lead to action. Talking about foods from other cultures can lead to cooking those foods, or to inviting international guests to our home. Talking about the environmental consequences of wasting food can lead to composting, eating green, using leftovers, or redistributing unused food. Talking about the economic disparities that limit access to healthy food in poor communities can lead to joining forces with food justice groups and to urban gardening. Any of these conversations can lead to raising money for social justice organizations through cooking or baking.

Dinner is like a small plot of land that can be seeded, fertilized, and coaxed to yield a series of crops. Dinner is a small plot of time that can be sowed to reap comfort, fun, play, and curiosity about the wider world, playful and meaningful conversation, and even action to change the world one meal at a time.

Notes

Chapter 2   What's So Great About Family Dinners?

1. B. Fiese and M. Schwartz, "Reclaiming the Family Table: Mealtimes and Child Health Well-Being," *Social Policy Report* 22(4) (2008): 3–16.
2. B. Sen, "The Relationship Between Frequency of Family Dinner and Adolescent Problem Behaviors After Adjusting for Other Family Characteristics," *Journal of Adolescence* 33 (2010): 187–196; M. E. Eisenberg, R. Olson, D. Neumark-Sztainer, M. Story, and L. H. Bearinger, "Correlations Between Family Meals and Psychosocial Well-Being Among Adolescents," *Archives of Pediatrics and Adolescent Medicine* 158 (2004): 792–796; J. Fulkerson, M. Story, A. Mellin, N. Leffert, D. Neumark-Sztainer, and S. French, "Family Dinner Meal Frequency and Adolescent Development: Relationships with Developmental Assets and High-Risk Behaviors," *Journal of Adolescent Health* 39(3) (2006): 337–345.
3. P. Steinglass, L. Bennett, S. J. Wolin, and D. Reiss, *The Alcoholic Family* (New York: Basic Books, 1987).
4. There are varying degrees of rigor and robustness in the research on family dinners. Any research that is correlational or cross-sectional

opens itself to criticism about causality. If, for example, dinners are *correlated* with positive outcomes like increased well-being and decreased substance abuse, it isn't the same as knowing whether having family dinners *causes* these positive behaviors in children. Some cross-sectional studies are improved by controlling for overarching variables. Still other studies are longitudinal, looking at more than one moment in time, a type of methodology that makes it easier to infer causality. The gold standard for research would be unethical to carry out—randomly assigning some families to eating dinner separately in bedrooms while watching TV, and assigning others to regular mealtimes in the kitchen as a family.

5. F. J. Elgar, W. Craig, and S. J. Trites, "Family Dinners, Communication, and Mental Health in Canadian Adolescents," *Journal of Adolescent Health* 52(4) (2013): 433–438; A. Meier and K. Musick, "Family Dinners and Adolescent Well-Being," California Center for Populations Research, online, working paper series, 1–33, June 2012.

6. D. Dickinson and P. Tabors, eds., *Beginning Literacy and Language: Young Children Learning at Home and School.* (Baltimore: Paul H. Brooks Publishing, 2002). The Home-School Study of Language and Literacy Development.

7. C. E. Snow and D. E. Beals, "Mealtime That Supports Literacy Development," *New Directions for Child and Adolescent Development* 111 (Spring 2006).

8. S. L. Hofferth and J. F. Sandberg, "How American Children Spend Their Time," *Journal of Marriage and the Family* 63 (2001): 295–308.

9. B. Fiese, "Family Matters: A Systems View of Family Effects on Children's Cognitive Health," *Environmental Effects on Cognitive Abilities*, ed. R. J. Sternberg and E. L. Grigorenko (Mahwah, NJ: Lawrence Erlbaum, 2000), 39–57.

10. G. H. Brody and D. L. Flor, "Maternal Psychological Functioning, Family Processes, and Child Adjustment in Rural, Single Parent, African American Families," *Developmental Psychology* 33 (1997): 1000–1011.

11. The National Center on Addiction and Substance Abuse at Columbia University (CASA), "The Importance of Family Dinners," 2003, 2007,

2009, 2010; retrieved from http://www.casacolumbia.org/templates/
Publications_Reports.askpx.

12. Fulkerson, Story, Meillin, Leffer, Neumark-Sztainer, and French, "Family Dinner Meal Frequency and Adolescent Development: Relationships with Developmental Assets and High-Risk Behaviors," 337–345; B. Sen, "The Relationship Between Frequency of Family Dinner and Adolescent Problem Behaviors After Adjusting for Other Family Characteristics," *Journal of Adolescence* 33 (2010): 187–196.

13. M. E. Eisenberg, R. E. Olson, D. Neumark-Sztainer, M. Story, and L. H. Bearinger, "Correlations Between Family Meals and Psychosocial Well-being Among Adolescents," *Archives of Pediatrics and Adolescent Medicine* 158 (2004): 792–796.

14. M. E. Eisenberg, D. Neumark-Sztainer, J. A. Fulkerson, and M. Story, "Family Meals and Substance Abuse: Is There a Long-Term Protective Association?" *Journal of Adolescent Health* 43 (2008): 145–151.

15. D. Neumark-Sztainer, M. E. Eisenberg, J. A. Fulkerson, M. Story, and N. Larson, "Family Meals and Disordered Eating in Adolescents," *Archive Pediatric and Adolescent Medicine* 162(21) (2008): 17–22.

16. D. Neumark-Sztainer, M. Wall, M. Story, and J. A. Fulkerson, "Are Family Meal Patterns Associated with Disordered Eating Behaviors Among Adolescents?" *Journal of Adolescent Health* 35 (2004): 350–359.

17. Fulkerson, Story, Mellin, Leffert, Neumark-Sztainer, and French, "Family Dinner Meal Frequency and Adolescent Development: Relationships with Developmental Assets and High-Risk Behaviors," 337–345.

18. S. Gable, Y. Chang, and J. Krull, "Television Watching and Frequency of Family Meals Are Predictive of Overweight Onset and Persistence in a National Sample of School-Aged Children," *Journal of the American Dietetic Association* 107 (2007): 53–61.

19. M. W. Gilman, S. L. Rifas-Shiman, A. L. Frazier, H. Rocket, C. A. Camargo, A. E. Feld, C. S. Berkey, and G. A. Colditz, "Family Dinner and Diet Quality Among Older Children and Adolescents," *Archives of Family Medicine* 9 (2000): 235–240. These findings were based on the children's own self-report of what they ate in the previous twenty-four

hours and were robust findings, even when household income, maternal employment, body mass index and physical activity were taken out of the equation.

20. M. S. Faith, K. S. Scanlon, L. L. Birch, L. S. Francis, and B. Sherry, "Parent-Child Feeding Strategies and Their Relationships to Child Eating and Weight Status," *Obesity Research* 12 (2004): 1711–1722.

21. M. P. Jacobs and B. H. Fiese, "Family Mealtime Interactions and Overweight Children with Asthma," *Journal of Pediatric Psychology* 32(1) (2007): 64–68.

22. S. Markson and B. Fiese, "Family Rituals as a Protective Factor for Children with Asthma," *Journal of Pediatric Psychology* 25(7) (2000): 471–479.

23. B. H. Fiese, M. A. Winter, and J. C. Botti, "The ABCs of Family Mealtimes: Observational Lessons for Promoting Healthy Outcomes for Children," *Child Development* 82(1) (2011): 144–151.

24. M. W. Gilman, S. L. Rifas-Shiman, A. L. Frazier, H. R. Rockett, C. A. Camargo, A. E. Field, C. S. Berkey, and G. A. Colditz, "Family Dinner Quality Among Older Children and Adolescents," *Archives of Family Medicine* 9(3) (2000): 235–240; T. M. Videon and C. K. Manning, "Influences on Adolescent Eating Patterns: The Importance of Family Meals," *Journal of Adolescent Health* 32 (2003): 365–373; J. A. Fulkerson, M. Y. Jubik, M. Story, L. Lytle, and C. Arcan, "Are There Nutritional and Other Benefits Associated with Family Meals Among At-Risk Youth?" *Journal of Adolescent Health* 45 (2009): 389–395.

25. N. I. Larson, D. Neumark-Sztainer, P. J. Hannan, and M. Story, "Family Meals During Adolescence Are Associated with Higher Diet Quality and Healthful Meal Patterns During Young Adulthood," *Journal of the American Dietetic Association* 107(8) (2007): 1502–1510.

26. CASA, 2010, file:///Users/annefishel/Downloads/The-importance-of-family-dinners-VI.pdf, accessed 9/3/14.

27. CASA, 2012, http://www.casacolumbia.org/addiction-research/reports/importance-of-family-dinners-2012, accessed 9/3/14.

28. C. Zoumas-Morse, C. L. Rock, E. L. Sobo, L. Marian, and M. L. Neuhouser, "Children's Patterns of Macronutrient Intake and Associations with Restaurant and Home Eating," *Journal of the American Dietetic Association* 101 (2001): 923–925.

29. R. Whiting, "Guidelines to Designing Therapeutic Rituals," in E. Imber-Black, J. Roberts, and R. Whiting (Eds.), *Rituals in Families and Family Therapy* (New York: Norton, 1988).

30. P. Steinglass, L. Bennett, S. J. Wolin, and D. Reiss, *The Alcoholic Family* (New York: Basic Books, 1987).

31. http://www.reelviews.net/php_review_template.php?identifier=186, accessed 9/3/14.

Chapter 3   One Size Dinner Doesn't Fit All Ages

1. J. Menella, M. Jagnow, and G. Beauchamp, "Prenatal and Postnatal Flavor Learning by Human Infants," *Pediatrics* 107(6) (2001): 88–94.

2. G. Beauchamp and J. Menella, "Early Flavor Learning and Its Impact on Later Feeding Behavior," *Journal of Pediatric Gastroenterology and Nutrition* 48 (2009): 25–30.

3. B. H. Fiese, *Family Routines and Rituals* (New Haven: Yale University Press, 2006).

4. H. Bante, M. Elliott, A. Harrod, and D. Haire-Joshu, "The Use of Inappropriate Feeding Practices by Rural Parents and Their Effect on Preschoolers' Fruit and Vegetable Preferences and Intake," *Journal of Nutrition Education and Behavior* 40(1) (2008): 28–33.

5. M. W. Gilman, S. L. Rifas-Shiman, A. L. Frazier, H. R. Rockett, C. A. Camargo, A. E. Field, C. S. Berkey, and G. A. Colditz, "Family Dinner and Diet Quality Among Older Children and Adolescents," *Archives of Family Medicine* 9(3) (2000): 235–240.

6. S. Hauser, S. Powers, and G. Noam, *Adolescents and Their Families: Paths of Ego Development* (New York: Free Press, 1991).

7. M. F. K. Fisher, *Serve It Forth* (New York: Macmillan Publishing Company, 1937).

Chapter 4   Tips for Healthy Eating

1. http://www.ers.usda.gov/topics/food-markets-prices/processing-marketing/new-products.aspx#.U_ycabxdVlw, accessed 8/26/14.

2. B. Wansink, *Mindless Eating: Why We Eat More Than We Think* (New York: Random House, 2010).

3. W. Willet, *Eat, Drink, and Be Healthy* (New York: Simon and Schuster, 2001), 27.

4. http://www.sciencedaily.com/.

5. C. Ogden and M. Carroll, "Prevalence of Obesity Among Children and Adolescents: United States, Trends 1963–1965 through 2007–2008," Centers for Disease Control, National Center for Health Statistics, June 2010; C. L. Ogden, M. D. Carroll, B. K. Kit, and K. M. Flegal, "Prevalence of Childhood and Adult Obesity in the United States, 2011–2012," *Journal of the American Medical Association* 311(8) (2014): 806–814.

6. M. Wabitsch, A. Moss, and K. Kromeyer-Hauschild, "Unexpected Plateauing of Childhood Obesity Rates in Developed Countries," http://www.biomedcentral.com/1741–7015/12/17.

7. Ibid.

8. B. N. Ogata and D. Hayes, "Position of Nutrition and Dietetics: Nutrition Guidance for Children Ages 2 to 11 Years Position Statement," *Journal of the Academy of Nutrition and Dietetics* 114(8) (2014): 1257–1276.

9. Position of the American Dietetic Association: Dietary Guidance for Healthy Children Ages 2–11 Years, *Journal of the American Dietetic Association* 104(7) (2004): 660–677.

10. S. Savage, J. O. Fisher, and L. L. Birch, "Parental Influence on Eating Behavior: Conception to Adolescence," *Journal of Law and Medical Ethics* 35(1) (2007): 22–34.

11. Michael Pollan, *In Defense of Food* (New York: Penguin Press, 2008).

12. Rachel Herz, That's Disgusting: Unraveling the Mysteries of Repulsion (New York: W. W. Norton, 2012).

13. L. J. Cooke, C. M. A. Haworth, and J. Wardle, "Genetic and Environmental Influences on Children's Food Neophobia," *American Journal of Clinical Nutrition* 86 (2007): 428–433.

14. Isobel Contento, Columbia University Teacher's College.

15. J. M. Berge, R. MacLehos, K. A. Loth, M. Eisenberg, M. M. Bucchianeri, and D. Neumark-Sztainer, "Parent Conversations About Healthful Eating and Weight: Associations with Adolescent Disordered Eating Behavior," *JAMA Pediatrics* 167(8) (2013): 746–753.

16. L. A. Francis and L. L. Birch, "Maternal Influences on Daughters' Restrained Eating Behavior," *Health Psychology* 24(6) (2005): 548–554.

17. S. A. Sullivan and L. L. Birch, "Pass the Sugar, Pass the Salt: Experience Dictates Preference," *Developmental Psychology* 26 (1990): 546–551.

18. Y. Martins, University of South Australia.

19. A. T. Galloway, L. M. Fiorito, L. A. Francis, and L. L. Birch, " 'Finish Your Soup': Counterproductive Effects of Pressuring Children to Eat on Intake and Affect," *Appetite* 46(3) (2006): 318–323.

20. J. O. Fisher and L. L. Birch, "Restricting Access to Palatable Foods Affects Children's Behavioral Response, Food Selection, and Intake," *American Journal of Clinical Nutrition* 69(6) (1999): 1264–1272.

21. Michael Pollan, *Food Rules* (New York: Penguin Press, 2011). I have given only a sampling of his eighty-three rules.

22. Marion Nestle, *What to Eat* (New York: North Point Press, 2006).

23. K. C. Copeland, P. Zeitler, M. Geffner, C. Guandalini, J. Higgins, K. Hirst, F. R. Kaufman, B. Linder, S. Marcovina, P. McGuigan, L. Pyle, W. Tamborlane, and S. Willi for the TODAY Study Group, "Characteristics of Adolescents and Youth with Recent-Onset Type 2 Diabetes: The TODAY Cohort at Baseline," *Journal of Clinical Endocrinology & Metabolism* 96 (2011): 159–167.

24. http://www.helpguide.org/life/healthy_diet_diabetes.htm, http://www.eatright.org/Public/content.aspx?id=6813.

25. J. Baio, "Prevalence of Autism Spectrum Disorder Among Children Aged 8 Years," Autism and Developmental Disabilities Monitoring Network, 11 sites, U.S., 2010. *Surveillance summaries*: March 28, 2014/63(SS02): 1–21. Accessed 4/9/14, http://www.cdc.gov/mmwr/preview/mmwrhtml/ss6302a1.htm?s_cid=ss6302a1_w.

26. S. M. Shore, *Beyond the Wall: Personal Experiences with Autism and Asperger Syndrome* (Shawnee Mission, KS: Autism Asperger Publishing Co., 2001).

27. Clinical details have been changed to protect the identity of the patient.

28. http://www.cdc.gov/nchs/data/databriefs/db121.htm, accessed 9/3/14.

29. http://www.foodallergy.org/document.doc?id=133.

30. http://www.foodallergy.org/tools-and-resources/managing-food
    -allergies/cooking-and-baking?.

Chapter 5   Play with Your Food

1. N. Chaudhari, A. M. Landin, and S. D. Roper, "A Metabotropic Glu-
   tamate Receptor Variant Functions as a Taste Receptor," *Nature Neu-
   roscience* 3 (2000): 113–119.

2. C. Bushdid, M. O. Magnasco, L. B. Vosshall, and A. Keller, "Humans
   Can Discriminate More Than 1 Trillion Olfactory Stimuli," *Science*
   343(6177) (2014): 1370–1372; www.sciencemag.org/content/343/6177/
   1370, accessed 8/26/14.

3. R. Schoenthaler, www.thefamilydinnerproject.org/family-blog/moving
   -beyond-picky-eating.

4. Richard Wrangham, *Catching Fire: How Cooking Made Us Human*
   (New York: Basic Books, 2010).

5. V. Rideout, U. Foehr, and D. Roberts, *Generation M2: Media in the
   Lives of 8- to 18-Year-Olds* (Menlo Park, CA: Henry J. Kaiser Family
   Foundation, 2010).

Chapter 6   Table Talk That Goes Beyond "How Was Your Day?"

1. M. Chouinard, "Analysis of the Childes Database," *Monographs of the
   Society for Research in Child Development* 72(1) (2007): 14–44.

2. http://www.thedigitalfamily.org/.

3. http://sites.gse.harvard.edu/making-caring-common/resources
   -publications/research-report, accessed 9/30/14. For more research
   and advice on raising ethical children.

4. Susan Dominus, "Table Talk: The New Family Dinner," *New York
   Times,* April 27, 2012.

5. M. P. Duke, R. Fivush, A. Lazarus, and J. Bohanek, "Of Ketchup and
   Kin: Dinnertime Conversations as a Major Source of Family Knowl-

edge, Family Adjustment, and Family Resilience," The Emory Center for Myth and Ritual in American Life, Working Paper No. 26, May 2003.

Chapter 7   Telling Stories to Promote Empathy, Self-Esteem, Resilience, and Enjoyment

1. M. P. Duke, A. Lazarus, and R. Fivush, "Knowledge of Family History as a Clinically Useful Index of Psychological Well-Being and Prognosis: A Brief Report," *Psychotherapy Theory, Research, Practice, Training* 45 (2008): 268–272.

2. R. Fivush, J. G. Bohanek, and M. Duke, "The Intergenerational Self: Subjective Perspective and Family History," Emory Center for Myth and Ritual in American Life, Working Paper No. 44, 2005.

3. C. E. Snow and D. E. Beals, "Mealtime Talk That Supports Literacy," *New Directions for Child and Adolescent Development,* no. 111 (2006): 51–66.

4. C. E. Snow, "Literacy and Language: Relationships During the Preschool Years," *Harvard Educational Review* 53 (1983): 165–189.

5. P. O. Tabors, C. E. Snow, and D. K. Dickenson, *Homes and Schools Together: Supporting Language and Literacy Development* (Baltimore: Brooks, 2001), 313–334.

6. R. Fivush, "Maternal Reminiscing Style and Children's Developing Understanding of Self and Emotion," *Clinical Social Work Journal* 35 (2007): 37–46.

7. C. Peterson, B. Jesso, and A. McCabe, *Journal of Child Language* 26(1) (1999): 49–67.

8. Ibid.

9. E. Reese, A. Bird, and G. Tripp, "Children's Self-Esteem and Moral Self: Links to Parent-Child Conversations About Emotion," *Social Development* 16: 460–478.

10. D. Laible, "Mother-Child Discourse in Two Contexts: Links with Child Temperament, Attachment Security, and Socioemotional Competence," *Developmental Psychology* 20 (2004): 979–992.

11. Duke, Fivus, Lazarus, and Bohanek, "Of Ketchup and Kin: Dinner-time Conversations as a Major Source of Family Knowledge, Family Adjustment, and Family Resilience."

12. A. Thorne, K. C. McLean, and A. Dasbach, "When Parents' Stories Go to Pot: Telling Personal Transgression to Teenage Kids," *Family Stories and the Life Course: Across Time and Generations*, ed. M. W. Pratt and B. H. Fiese (Mahwah, NJ: Lawrence Erlbaum Associates, 2004).

13. Sonia Sotomayer, *My Beloved World* (New York: Knopf, 2013).

14. D. McAdams, "Generativity and the Narrative Ecology of Family Life," *Family Stories and the Life Course: Across Time and Generations*, ed. M. W. Pratt and B. H. Fiese (Mahweh, NJ: Lawrence Erlbaum Associates, 2004).

15. P. Gould, "Telling Stories and Getting Acquainted: How Age Matters," *Family Stories and the Life Course: Across Time and Generations*, ed. M. W. Pratt and B. H. Fiese (Mahwah, NJ: Lawrence Erlbaum Associates, 2004).

16. J. Norris, S. Kuiack, and M. W. Pratt, "As Long as They Go Back Down the Driveway at the End of the Day: Stories of the Satisfactions and Challenges of Grandparenthood," *Family Stories and the Life Course: Across Time and Generations*, ed. M. W. Pratt and B. H. Fiese (Mahwah, NJ: Lawrence Erlbaum Associates, 2004).

17. D. McAdams, J. Reynolds, M. Lewis, A. Patten, and P. Bowman, "When Bad Things Turn Good and Good Things Turn Bad: Sequences of Redemption and Contamination in Life Narrative and Their Relation to Psychosocial Adaptation in Midlife Adults and in Students," *Personality and Social Psychology Bulletin* 27(4) (2001): 474–485.

18. Laurie Colwin, *Home Cooking* (New York: Knopf, 1988); Laurie Colwin, *More Home Cooking: A Writer Returns to the Kitchen* (New York: Harper Collins, 1993).

Chapter 8   Lessons Learned from The Family Dinner Project

1. Thefamilydinnerproject.org.

2. Shelly London, Bob Stains, Lynn Barendsen, Ashley Sandvi, Wendy Fischman, Jono Reduker, Mary Reilly, Laura Chasin, and I. Other

people have joined the team over the past four years: Amy Yelin, Joanna Gallagher, Amy Burton, Grace Taylor, John Sarrouf, Charlotte Svirsky, Kelly Johnston, Alyssa Wickham, Paromita De, Dave Joseph, Bri DeRosa. And still others have been consultants to us: Nico Mele, Morra Aarons-Mele, Christine Koh, Debbie Halpern, Howard Gardner. We have received help and guidance from the Public Conversations Project in Watertown, MA, and from The Good Project at the Harvard Graduate School of Education School. Shelly London first conceived of The Family Dinner Project while an inaugural fellow in Harvard's Advanced Leadership Initiative. While at Harvard, she worked with partners, students, and professors to develop a multifaceted, multimedia program to promote ethical thinking and conversation about ethics. Since everyday ethics—talk about the choices we make as individuals and the way we treat each other every day—start at home, family dinners are a prime time to help families come together to talk about these issues. As Shelly conducted research on family dinners during her fellowship, she connected with a group of people who became the founding members of The Family Dinner Project team.

3. Not their real names.
4. Not their real names.

Chapter 9   Dinner as a Laboratory for Change

1. The names and other identifying features have been changed for all the clinical examples offered in this chapter.
2. Patricia L. Papernow, *Surviving and Thriving in Stepfamily Relationships: What Works and What Doesn't* (New York: Routledge, 2013).
3. http://thefamilydinnerproject.org/food-for-thought/steps-to-ease-dinner-stress-for-stepfamilies/.
4. P. Rauch and A. Muriel, *Raising an Emotionally Healthy Child When a Parent Is Sick* (New York: McGraw-Hill, 2006).
5. R. Basson, "Women's Difficulties with Low Sexual Desire, Sexual Avoidance, and Sexual Aversion," *Handbook of Clinical Sexuality for*

Mental Health Professionals, second edition, ed. S. B. Levine, C. B. Risen, and S. E. Althof (New York: Routledge, 2011).

Chapter 10   Extending the Dinner Table to the Wide World

1. J. Billing and P. W. Sherman, "Antimicrobial Functions of Spices: Why Some Like It Hot," *The Quarterly Review of Biology* 73(1) (1998): 3–49.
2. http://www.nrdc.org/food/files/wasted-food-ip.pdf.
3. K. Moreland, S. Wing, A. D. Roux, and C. Poule, "Neighborhood Characteristics Associated with the Location of Food Stores and Food Service Places," *American Journal of Preventive Medicine* 22(1) (2002): 23–29.
4. U.S. Department of Agriculture (USDA) 2009 access to affordable and nutritious food: Measuring and understanding food deserts and their consequences. Washington, DC: Economic Research Service.
5. Tristram Stewart, *Waste: Uncovering the Global Food Scandal* (New York: W. W. Norton, 2009).
6. Phone conversation with author, February 27, 2014.
7. TED Talk, TedxDirigo, September 2011, https://www.ted.com/talks/roger_doiron_my_subversive_garden_plot, accessed 2/25/14.
8. Conversation with David Gass.
9. http://www.farmtoschool.org/.
10. http://edibleschoolyard.org/node/102, accessed 9/30/14.
11. http://www.nrdc.org/food/files/wasted-food-ip.pdf.
12. Ibid.
13. http://www.fao.org.
14. http://www.nrdc.org/food/files/wasted-food-ip.pdf.
15. http://worldnews.nbcnews.com/_news/2013/06/05/18780415-wasting-food-is-like-stealing-from-the-poor-says-pope?lite.
16. http://www.foodrecoverynetwork.org/;   http://www.thinkeatsave.org/; http://www.feeding5k.org/gleaning.php.
17. http://www.nrdc.org/food/expiration-dates.asp.
18. http://england.lovefoodhatewaste.com/hints-and-tips.

19. http://england.lovefoodhatewaste.com/content/food-waste-recycling -what-do-food-you-cant-eat.

20. http://www.nrdc.org/globalWarming/files/eatgreenfs_feb2010.pdf.

21. http://randd.defra.gov.uk/Document.aspx?Document=EV02007 _4601_FRP.pdf.

22. http://www.nrdc.org/globalWarming/files/eatgreenfs_feb2010.pdf.

23. Clinton Global Initiative: Challah for Hunger, https://www.youtube .com/watch?v=5Xe6KQmzaLw, accessed 9/3/14

24. Phone conversation with author, January 2014.

Resources

About Children Ages 2-6

Cooke, L. J., C. M. A. Haworth, and J. Wardle. "Genetic and Environmental Influences on Children's Food Neophobia." *American Journal of Clinical Nutrition* 86 (2007): 428–433.

Dickinson, D., and P. Tabors, eds. *Beginning Literacy and Language: Young Children Learning at Home and School.* Baltimore: Paul H. Brooks Publishing, 2002. The Home-School Study of Language and Literacy Development.

Gable, S., Y. Chang, and J. Krull. "Television Watching and Frequency of Family Meals Are Predictive of Overweight Onset and Persistence in a National Sample of School-Aged Children." *Journal of the American Dietetic Association* 107 (2007): 53–61.

Galloway, A. T., L. M. Fiorito, L. A. Francis, and L. L. Birch. " 'Finish Your Soup': Counterproductive Effects of Pressuring Children to Eat on Intake and Affect." *Appetite* 46(3) (2006): 318–323.

Menella, J., M. Jagnow, and G. Beauchamp. "Prenatal and Postnatal Flavor Learning by Human Infants." *Pediatrics* 107(6) (2001): 88–94.

Snow, C. E., and D. E. Beals. "Mealtime That Supports Literacy Development." *New Directions for Child and Adolescent Development* 111 (Spring 2006).

Sullivan, S. A., and L. L. Birch. "Pass the Sugar, Pass the Salt: Experience Dictates Preference." *Developmental Psychology* 26 (1990): 546–551.

About Children Ages 6–12

Brody, G. H., and D. L. Flor. "Maternal Psychological Functioning, Family Processes, and Child Adjustment in Rural, Single Parent, African American Families." *Developmental Psychology* 33 (1997): 1000–1011.

Faith, M. S., K. S. Scanlon, L. L. Birch, L. S. Francis, and B. Sherry. "Parent-Child Feeding Strategies and Their Relationships to Child Eating and Weight Status." *Obesity Research* 12 (2004): 1711–1722.

Fiese, B., and M. Schwartz. "Reclaiming the Family Table: Mealtimes and Child Health Well-Being." *Social Policy Report* 22(4) (2008): 3–16.

Fiese, B. H., M. A. Winter, and J. C. Botti. "The ABCs of Family Meal-Times: Observational Lessons for Promoting Healthy Outcomes for Children." *Child Development* 82(1) (2011): 144–151.

Hofferth, S. L., and J. F. Sandberg. "How American Children Spend Their Time." *Journal of Marriage and the Family* 63 (2001): 295–308.

Jacobs, M. P., and B. H. Fiese. "Family Mealtime Interactions and Overweight Children with Asthma." *Journal of Pediatric Psychology* 32(1) (2007): 64–68.

About Teens

Eisenberg, M. E., D. Neumark-Sztainer, J. A. Fulkerson, and M. Story. "Family Meals and Substance Abuse: Is There a Long-Term Protective Association?" *Journal of Adolescent Health* 43 (2008): 145–151.

Eisenberg, M. E., R. Olson, D. Neumark-Sztainer, M. Story, and L. H. Bearinger. "Correlations Between Family Meals and Psychosocial Well-Being Among Adolescents." *Archives of Pediatrics and Adolescent Medicine* 158 (2004): 792–796.

Fulkerson, J., M. Story, A. Mellin, N. Leffert, D. Neumark-Sztainer, and S. French. "Family Dinner Meal Frequency and Adolescent Development: Relationships with Developmental Assets and High-Risk Behaviors." *Journal of Adolescent Health* 39(3) (2006): 337–345.

Gilman, M. W., S. L. Rifas-Shiman, A. L. Frazier, H. R. Rockett, C. A. Camargo, A. E. Field, C. S. Berkey, and G. A. Colditz. "Family Dinner Quality Among Older Children and Adolescents." *Archives of Family Medicine* 9(3) (2000): 235–240.

National Center on Addiction and Substance Abuse at Columbia University (CASA). "The Importance of Family Dinners," 2003, 2007, 2009, 2010. Retrieved from http://www.casacolumbia.org/templates/Publications_Reports.askpx.

Neumark-Sztainer, D., M. E. Eisenberg, J. A. Fulkerson, M. Story, and N. Larson. "Family Meals and Disordered Eating in Adolescents." *Archive Pediatric and Adolescent Medicine* 162(21) (2008): 17–22.

Sen, B., "The Relationship Between Frequency of Family Dinner and Adolescent Problem Behaviors After Adjusting for Other Family Characteristics." *Journal of Adolescence* 33 (2010): 187–196.

Videon, T. M., and C. K. Manning. "Influences on Adolescent Eating Patterns: The Importance of Family Meals." *Journal of Adolescent Health* 32 (2003).

Other Suggested Resources

Duke, M. P., R. Fivush, A. Lazarus, and J. Bohanek. "Of Ketchup and Kin: Dinner-time Conversations as a Major Source of Family Knowledge, Family Adjustment, and Family Resilience." The Emory Center for Myth and Ritual in American Life. Working Paper No. 26. May 2003.

The Family Dinner Project: http://thefamilydinnerproject.org/.

Fiese, B. H. *Family Routines and Rituals.* New Haven: Yale University Press, 2006.

Herz, Rachel. That's Disgusting: Unraveling the Mysteries of Repulsion. New York: W. W. Norton, 2012.

Making Caring Common Project: http://bit.ly/1E1Uil4.

Nestle, M. *What to Eat.* New York: North Point Press, 2006.

Pollan, M. *Food Rules.* New York: Penguin Press, 2011.

———. *In Defense of Food.* New York: Penguin Press, 2008.

Stewart, T. *Waste: Uncovering the Global Food Scandal.* New York: W. W. Norton, 2009.

Wansink, B. *Mindless Eating: Why We Eat More Than We Think.* New York: Random House, 2010.

Willet, W. *Eat, Drink, and Be Healthy.* New York: Simon & Schuster, 2001.

Cookbooks and Food Writing to Inspire Children and Parents

Aaron, F. *What Chefs Feed Their Kids.* Guilford, CT: Globe Pequot Press, 2012.

Colwin, L. *Home Cooking.* New York: Knopf, 1988.

———. *More Home Cooking: A Writer Returns to the Kitchen.* New York: Harper-Collins, 1993.

Fisher, M. F. K. *Serve It Forth.* New York: Macmillan, 1937.

Hamilton, G. *Bread, Bones, and Butter.* New York: Random House, 2012.

Katzen, M. *Honest Pretzels: And 64 Other Amazing Recipes.* Berkeley, CA: Tricycle Press, 2009.

Katzen, M. *Pretend Soup and Other Real Recipes: A Cookbook for Preschoolers and Up.* Berkeley, CA: Tricycle Press, 1994.

Reichl, R. *Tender at the Bone: Growing Up at the Table.* New York: Broadway, 1999.

Rosenstrach. J. *Dinner: A Love Story.* New York: HarperCollins, 2012.

Sampson, S., and C. Tremblay. *ChopChop: The Kids' Guide to Cooking Real Food with Your Family.* New York: Simon & Schuster, 2013.

Samuelsson, M. *Yes, Chef.* New York: Random House, 2012.

Young, K., ed. *The Hungry Ear: Poems of Food and Drink.* New York: Bloomsbury, 2012.

Index

adolescents
  academic performance
    of, 17
  conversing with, 116
  food play for, 97–102
  identity exploration by,
    37–38, 45, 165
  level of involvement in
    family dinners, 24,
    38–40
  meal preparation by, 39
  mental health of, 12,
    17–18
  music preferences of, 93
  parental relationships of,
    6, 14
  physical health of, 19
African Americans, 17, 183
alcoholism, 12, 129
allergies, 75–76, 178
Allison, Jay, 111
American Dietetic
  Association, 51
antibacterial foods, 181–182
anxiety, 19, 74, 128
appetite stimulation, 45,
  175
Asian chicken wings
  (recipe), 35, 37

assisted living facilities,
  44–45
asthma, 19, 74
autism spectrum disorder
  (ASD), 73–75

Banana Boats (recipe), 86
Barendsen, Lynn, 94
*Battle Hymn of the Tiger
  Mother* (Chua), 116
Billing, Jennifer, 181
binge drinking, 17
binge eating, 55
Black Bean Burgers (recipe),
  60–62
Blood, Bones and Butter
  (Hamilton), 90
blood sugar, 71
Bluefish with Schmear
  (recipe), 66
Blue Plate Special
  (Christenson), 90
bread, 65, 82, 189, 195–197
Bread and Jam for Frances
  (Hoban), 88
breast-feeding, 25–26

calorie requirements, 49
cancer, 52

carbohydrates, 71, 72, 181
carbon footprint, 182, 192
celiac disease, 76
Challah for Hunger (CfH),
  194–197
Challah for Hunger Bread
  (recipe), 196–197
cheese, 62, 63, 84, 189
Chez Panisse, 186
Chicken Soup (recipe),
  64–66
children. See adolescent,
  preschool-age children,
  school-age children,
  young adults
children's books, 88
ChopChop (Sampson), 32
Chua, Amy, 116
Clinton, Bill, 194
color
  of foods for illness, 78–82
  memory of, 89
  and nutritional value, 52,
    62, 70
  playing with, 78–82
Colwin, Laurie, 29, 90,
  133–134
Comfort Me with Apples
  (Reichl), 90

composting, 185, 191–192
conflict, managing, 33,
    38–39, 108–109
conversation. *See also*
    storytelling
  and autism spectrum
    disorder, 74
  food as stimulant for, 8
  "How was your day?,"
    103
  intellectual benefits of,
    7, 15
  setting guidelines for, 109,
    145
  and slower eating, 21
  techniques for deepening,
    106–108
  techniques for engaging
    children in, 104–106
  therapeutic role of, 8–9
  topics for, 39, 116–118
Conversation Starters in a
    Jar game, 115–116
cookies, 79–80, 83, 87–88
cooking
  to eat well, 58–59
  by elderly people, 44–45
  with fire, 85–86
  and food pickiness, 55
  for fund-raising, 193–194
  games involving, 94–95
  improvising in, 66–68,
    77–78
  music during, 78, 93–94
  with preschool children,
    27–32, 70
  with school-age children,
    35, 36–37, 70
  as sensual, 102
  by teens, 39
  therapeutic value of,
    161–163
Crane, Claire, 184
Crepes (recipe), 36–37

dairy foods, 56, 57, 61, 72,
    75, 76
Dana-Farber Cancer
    Institute, 193
Delicious Revolution, 186
depression
  and family stories, 128
  and food cravings, 181
  among teens, 12, 18

diabetes, 52, 70, 71–73,
    130–131
diet
  fads in, 50
  recommendations for, 51,
    56–57, 71
  special requirements for,
    69–76
  Western, 52, 57
dieting, 55, 70
dinner guests, 39, 177–180
dinner parties
  for families, 155–157
  for fund-raising, 193–194
  for international guests,
    177–180
divorce, 170–171
Doiron, Roger, 183–184
Duke Center for Eating
    Disorders, 56

eating disorders, 6, 18, 55
Edible Schoolyard, 186
elderly people, meals for,
    44–45
*The Elephant Walk
    Cookbook,* 68
emotional development
  and age level, 52
  and game playing, 110
  and storytelling, 123, 125,
    128
Empanadas from Cleo
    (recipe), 153
empathy, 125–127
empty nesters, 40–41, 166,
    168–170
environmentalism, 182–183,
    191, 192–193
Ephron, Nora, 95
Epicurious.com, 39, 72
explanatory talk, 15–16
exposure therapy, 75

fajitas, 147, 148, 150
family
  defining, 10
  food preferences
    within, 52
  healthy, characteristics
    of, 24
family dinner. *See also*
    cooking; meals
  committing to, 140–141

conflict during, 38–39,
    108–109
  conversation during (*see*
    conversation)
  and divorce, 170–171
  elderly people at, 44–45
  and empty nesters, 40–41,
    168–170
  and family connection,
    13–14, 19, 20
  frequency of, 10–11, 13, 16
  games during, 32,
    109–116
  goal setting for, 141, 142,
    144, 145
  guests at, 39, 177–180
  intellectual benefits of,
    15–17
  location of, 92
  manners at, 108
  and marriage, 166–168
  mental health benefits of,
    17–18
  multiple courses in, 32
  for multiple families,
    155–157
  music at, 40, 93–94
  nostalgia for, 42, 45,
    89–90
  nutritional value of,
    20–21, 49
  and parental illness,
    172–173
  physical health benefits
    of, 18–19
  portable, 35, 157
  power struggles
    during, 33
  as relationship changers,
    159–165, 173–175
  relaxation techniques
    used during, 56
  as ritual, 21–23, 27, 143,
    145
  routines in, 34–35, 74,
    170, 173
  scheduling of, 39
  seating arrangements for,
    92–93
  and stepparents, 171–172
  storytelling during (*see*
    storytelling)
  technology use during,
    39, 109, 126

therapeutic value of,
  6–7, 8, 9, 12, 13, 22,
  165–166, 176
Family Dinner Project, The,
  community dinners
    hosted by, 87, 93,
    145–150
  conversation topics from,
    117
  dietary recommendations
    of, 57
  Food, Fun and
    Conversation: 4 Weeks
    to Better Family
    Dinners program, 149,
    154, 157–158
  formation of, 9, 139–140
  foundational ideas for,
    140–143
  functions of, 10, 139, 140
  games suggested by, 110,
    111, 112, 149
  pilot families for, 143–145
  recipes from, 150, 154–
    155
  teaching children about
    food, 71
  website for, 115, 157
  workshops held by,
    151–155
family history, 104, 119–120,
  128–132
family identity, 34, 120, 128
farmers' markets, 70, 192
Farm to School programs,
  186
fast food, 51, 58–59, 71, 182
fats, dietary, 49, 51, 52, 56,
  71, 72
Feedback (organization),
  183
Feeding America Food
  Bank Locator, 190
fermenting, 99–100
fire, cooking with, 85–86
fish, 65, 66, 67, 75, 189
Fisher, M. F. K., 45
Fish Sauce (recipe), 44
Fish Tacos (recipe), 100–101
food. See also fast food;
  meals; restaurant
  meals; specific foods
    access to, 71, 182–183, 188
    allergies to, 75–76, 178

centrality of, 143, 198
colors of, 52, 62, 70,
  78–82, 181
complaining about, 109
conversation about, 8,
  117–118
experimentation with, 40,
  43, 84, 98
expiration dates of, 189,
  190
in family identity, 34
forbidden, 56, 70
freezing, 65, 189
healthy, for children,
  18–19, 184–186
to instigate storytelling,
  133–134
for invalids, 180–182
to keep on hand, 61
locally grown, 192
marketing of, 29, 34, 35,
  49, 50, 70
memories of, 89–91
as metaphor, 175–176
pickiness about (see picky
  eating)
pickled/fermented, 97–100
playing with, 7–8, 32–33,
  77–102
poems about, 89
portion sizes of, 57, 190
preferences, 26, 27, 38,
  52–58, 67–68, 73
processed, 52, 57
quick-to-prepare, 58–69
refusal of, 25, 33, 52,
  127–128
as relaxation device, 20
as sensory experience, 44,
  45, 82–85
shopping for, 49–50
symbolism of, 21–22
texture of, 55–56, 73
in utero, 25
food banks, 189, 190
food coloring paintings,
  80–81
food crop diversity, 52
food fads, 50, 52
Food for Free, 195–196
food justice, 182–190,
  194–197
food memoirs, 90
Food Rules (Pollan), 57, 185

food waste, 183, 186–190,
  195–196
Food Word game, 114–115
Ford School (Lynn, MA),
  184, 185
Francis I, Pope, 188
freegans, 183
freezing food, 65, 189
Frittatas (recipe), 60
fruit
  children's preferences for,
    55
  as dietary requirement,
    51, 56
  in family dinners vs.
    restaurants, 49
  growing, 187–188
  health benefits of, 52, 70
  storing, 189
Fruit and Vegetable game,
  113
Fruit and Yogurt Parfaits
  (recipe), 157

games
  and dinner conversation,
    103
  with food, 94–95
  during meals, 32,
    109–116, 144, 149
  with music, 94
  storytelling, 125
gardening, 183–187
Gass, David, 184–185
global citizenship, 177, 183,
  198
gluten, 76
Goodman, Ellen, 50
grains, 52, 56, 58, 61, 71
grandparents, 22, 26, 106,
  129, 132, 151–155
Green Eggs and Ham
  (Seuss), 88
Green Sauce (recipe),
  134–135
Guacamole (recipe),
  155–156
Guess That Emotion game,
  110–111
Guess the Title game,
  111–112

Haugen, Jen, 75
Hazan, Marcella, 78

hearing, sense of, 111
Heartburn (Ephron), 95
heart disease, 52
Higglety-Pigglety game,
    113–114
Hispanics, 183
holidays, 74, 89, 90, 117, 152,
    178–179, 180
Home Cooking (Colwin),
    29, 90
Honest Pretzels (Katzen), 32
Hot Chocolate Sauce
    (recipe), 92
How Well Do You Know
    Me? game, 114

Ice Cream Cake (recipe), 91
illness, 172–173, 180–182
In Defense of Food (Pollan),
    57
infants, 25–26, 45, 51
international guests,
    177–180
invalid food, 180–182
Iron Chef game, 94–95

jook, 34, 181
Jook Adaptation (recipe),
    68–69
Joy of Cooking
    (Rombauer), 36

Katzen, Mollie, 32
khichdi, 181

lactose intolerance, 72, 75, 76
language
    development of, 15
    playing with, 88–89
Lasagna, Easy (recipe),
    154–155
Lee, Ang, 22
leftovers, 63–66, 153, 190
*The Lion, the Witch and the
    Wardrobe* (Lewis), 88
Little House in the Big Woods
    (Wilder), 88
London, Shelly, 9
low-income families, 19, 182
Lukas, Geoff, 97–98

manners, 108
Marina's Pasta with Shrimp
    and Clams (recipe), 41

marriage, 44, 167–168
Mary Poppins (Travers), 88
Massachusetts General
    Hospital, 4, 7, 71, 85,
    173
Mayo Clinic Center for
    Innovation, 147
Meal-in-Bowl Salad, 62–63
meals. *See also* family
    dinners
    allowing children to
        choose, 33–34, 57
    go-to, 59–62
    healthy, 49–52, 70
    at holidays, 74, 89, 90,
        152, 178–179, 180
    home-cooked, 4, 22, 42,
        144, 178
    from other cultures,
        39, 40
    repurposing, 63–66
    in restaurants, 20, 49, 51
    scientific research on,
        12–13
    and special diets, 69–76
    vs. snacking, 58
meat
    restricting consumption
        of, 57, 192–193
    storing, 65, 189
    umami taste of, 84
mental health benefits
    of family dinner(s), 17–18
    of family stories, 128
    of redemptive stories, 132
Meringue Cookies (recipe),
    87–88
Mindfulness game, 111
Muffins (recipe), 124
music
    for holidays, 89
    selected for dinner, 40
    while cooking, 78, 93–94
music lyric games, 115
My Beloved World
    (Sotomayor), 130
MyPlate.gov, 56–57, 70

Name That Tune game,
    115
narrative talk, 15–16,
    122–123. *See also*
    storytelling
Nestle, Marion, 52, 58

nutrition
    in family dinners, 18, 19,
        20, 49
    and home-grown food,
        185–186
    scientific research on,
        50–51
    for seniors, 44
nuts, 61, 71, 72, 75, 76

Obama, Michelle, 56
Obama family, 110, 183
obesity
    among children, 12, 18,
        19, 51, 70
    curbing, 184, 186
    rise in, 52
O'Donnell, Ellen, 71–73
Omar's Café, 146, 147, 149
Origami Dumplings
    (recipe), 29, 30–31

Papernow, Patricia, 171,
    172
parents
    of adolescents, 38
    and child obesity, 19
    children's relationships
        with, 20
    divorced, 170–172
    as eating examples, 55, 68,
        70, 84
    as family dinner
        facilitators, 141–143
    and food choices, 52
    illness of, 172–173
    responsibility for feeding,
        25–26, 58
    and storytelling, 105,
        122–123, 131–132
    teaching manners, 108
    workshops for, 151–155
pasta, 41, 61, 65, 67, 72
Pesto (recipe), 67
physical activity, 51
pickled foods, 97–100
Pickled Sungold Tomatoes
    (recipe), 98–99
picky eating, 27, 33, 52–56,
    67–68, 73, 127–128
pizza, 35, 72
Pizza (recipe), 156
play
    with food, 32–33, 77–102

games, 32, 94–95, 103, 109–116, 125
storytelling as, 121
Play Dough, 95–96
Pollan, Michael, 52, 57, 58, 185
portion sizes, 57
pregnancy, 12, 17, 25
preschool-age children
conversing with, 107
empathy development in, 125–127
food play for, 95–97
food preferences of, 26, 27, 54–58, 73
intellectual benefits of family dinner for, 15–16
level of involvement in family dinner, 24, 32, 57
meal preparation with, 27–32, 45, 70
mealtime games for, 110–113
nutrition for, 51
physical benefits of family dinner for, 18
power struggles with, 33
storytelling for, 120–125
Pretend Soup (Katzen), 32
Pretzels (recipe), 82–83
Price, Lisa, 89
processed food, 52, 57
protein, 56, 71
public health programs, 51
purging, 55

quick food, 58–69

Rauch, Paula, 173
reading skills, 12, 15, 16, 121–122
recipes
Asian Chicken Wings, 37
Banana Boats, 86
Black Bean Burgers, 60–62
Bluefish with Schmear, 66
Challah for Hunger Bread, 196–197
Chicken Soup, 64–66
Crepes, 36–37
Easy Lasagna, 154–155

Empanadas from Cleo, 153
Fajitas, 150
Fish Sauce, 44
Fish Tacos, 100–101
Frittatas, 60
Fruit and Yogurt Parfaits, 157
Green Sauce, 134–135
Guacamole, 155–156
Hot Chocolate Sauce, 92
Ice Cream Cake, 91
Jook Adaptation, 68–69
Marina's Pasta with Shrimp and Clams, 41
Meal-in-Bowl Salad, 62–63
Meringue Cookies, 87–88
Muffins, 124
Origami Dumplings, 30–31
Pesto, 67
Pickled Sungold Tomatoes, 98–99
Pizza, 156
Play Dough, 95–96
Pretzels, 82–83
Roasted Chicken, 63–64
Soap, 96
Sour Cucumbers, 99–100
Spring Rolls, Hoi An Style, 43–44
Sugar Cookies, 79–80
Sugar Water for Brighter Chalk, 96–97
Sushi Birthday Cake, 81–82
Tomato Bread Soup, 190–191
Vegetable Soup, 53–54
Whipped Cream with Berries, 150–151
refrigerator practices, 61, 189
restaurant meals, 20, 49, 51
rickets, 51
rituals
developing, 27, 29, 39
at family dinners, 143, 145
functions of, 21–23
Roasted Chicken (recipe), 63–64

Rose and Thorn game, 110
Roth, Caryn, 195

salads, 62–63, 78
Sampson, Sally, 32
sandwiches, 54, 83
Sarrouf, John, 71, 152, 153, 154
Satter, Ellen, 58
schmears, 66, 67
Schoenthaler, Robin, 85
school-age children
conversing with, 104–108
food play for, 97–102
food preferences of, 54–58, 73
intellectual benefits of family dinner for, 16–17
level of involvement in family dinner, 33–35, 57
meal preparation with, 35, 36–37, 45, 70
mealtime games for, 113–116
nutrition for, 51
physical benefits of family dinner for, 18–19
storytelling for, 128–129
Science Daily, 50
self-esteem, 12, 18, 120, 123, 128
sexuality
food metaphors in, 175–176
among teens, 17
Sherman, Paul, 181
Shore, Stephen, 73
Singer, Carol, 74–75
single-parent families, 19, 170–171
single people, healthy eating by, 44
smell (sense of), 44, 45, 85, 111
smoking, 17
s'mores, 86
snack foods, 49, 51, 56, 58, 70
Snow, Catherine, 16
Soap (recipe), 96
social justice issues, 182–190, 194–197
Sofra (restaurant), 97

soft drinks, 49, 51
Sotomayor, Sonia, 130–131
soup, 53–56, 64–66, 68–69,
    181, 190–191
Sour Cucumbers (recipe),
    99–100
Spring Rolls, Hoi An Style
    (recipe), 42, 43–44
stepfamilies, 171–172
Story Corps, 132
storytelling
    about day's events, 120
    about family history, 104,
        119–120, 128–131
    about food, 133–134
    function of, 120, 121
    as game, 125
    instigating, 132–133, 135
    with lessons, 127–128
    and memory, 89–90
    by parents, 131–132
    for preschool children,
        120–122, 123–125
    to promote empathy,
        125–127
    and reading skill, 15
    for school-age children,
        128–129
    teaching, 122–123
Strega Nona (dePaola), 88
Stuart, Tristram, 183
substance abuse, 12, 17, 18
sugar, 51, 52, 57, 71, 72
Sugar Cookies (recipe),
    79–80
Sugar Water for Brighter
    Chalk (recipe), 96–97
supermarkets
    as classrooms, 76

    product choices at, 49
    product placement at,
        57, 70
    scavenger hunts at, 71
Sushi Birthday Cake
    (recipe), 81–82
Swick, Susan, 28, 30

tacos, 35, 100–101
Taliaferro, Frances,
    133–134
Taliaferro, Lee, 133
taste (sense of), 44, 45,
    83–84, 89
Taylor, Grace, 71
teenagers. See adolescents
television
    as detrimental to health,
        51
    food advertised on, 34, 35
    during meals, 18, 40
Thumbs Up to the Chef
    game, 144
Tomato Bread Soup
    (recipe), 190–191
Troekel, Matt, 30
Two Truths and a Tall Tale
    game, 111, 149

Uchida, Mai, 80–81
U.S. Department of
    Agriculture
    (USDA), 56

vegetables
    children's consumption
        of, 51
    children's preferences
        for, 55

    and diabetes, 71
    as dietary requirement, 56
    in family dinners vs.
        restaurants, 49
    growing, 187–188
    health benefits of, 52, 70
    storing, 189
Vegetable Soup (recipe),
    53–54
vegetarianism, 6, 38, 40,
    164–165
The Very Hungry Caterpillar
    (Carle), 88
Vilsack, Tom, 56
vocabulary
    improving through
        conversation, 7, 15, 16
    improving through
        storytelling, 121,
        122–123

Waters, Alice, 186
WCAI radio, 111
whipped cream, 86–87
Whipped Cream with
    Berries (recipe),
    150–151
whole grains, 58, 71
Winkelman, Eli, 194
World Environment Day,
    188
Would You Rather game,
    112–113

Yes, Chef (Samuelsson), 90
young adults, 42–43, 45

Zimmerman, Carly, 194,
    197

About the Author

Anne K. Fishel, Ph.D., is an Associate Professor of Psychology, part-time, at the Harvard Medical School and Director of the Family and Couples Therapy Program at Massachusetts General Hospital in Boston, where she has won many teaching prizes from psychiatry residents and psychology interns. She also has a private practice focusing on clinical supervision and individual, couples, and family therapy.

Dr. Fishel is a cofounder of The Family Dinner Project, a nonprofit group that works online and in person to help families overcome the obstacles that get in the way of family dinners. She speaks, consults, and publishes widely on a range of issues to do with families and couples.

A magna cum laude graduate of Harvard University, she earned her doctorate in clinical psychology at the University of North Carolina in Chapel Hill.

Dr. Fishel is the author of *Treating the Adolescent in Family Therapy: A Developmental and Narrative Approach* (Jason Aronson, 1999). She writes a blog on Psychologytoday.com, "The Digital Family," and has also blogged about family issues for NPR and PBS. She is an editor for the *Harvard Review of Psychiatry* and *Couple and Family Psychology: Research and Practice*. She lives outside Boston with her husband and is the mother of two young adult sons.